Innovation and Industrial Leadership:
Lessons from Pharmaceuticals

By

Fabio Pammolli and Massimo Riccaboni

"Data before analysis. Analysis before policy or prescription."

—Simon Kuznets

Pammolli, Fabio and Riccaboni, Massimo, *Innovation and Industrial Leadership: Lessons from Pharmaceuticals* (Washington, D.C.: Center for Transatlantic Relations, Johns Hopkins University, 2007).

Center for Transatlantic Relations
American Consortium on EU Studies
EU Center of Excellence Washington D.C.
The Paul H. Nitze School of Advanced International Studies
The Johns Hopkins University
1717 Massachusetts Ave., NW, Suite 525
Washington, D.C. 20036
Tel. (202) 663-5880
Fax (202) 663-5879
Email: transatlantic@jhu.edu
http://transatlantic.sais-jhu.edu

ISBN 10: 0-9788821-4-8
ISBN 13: 978-0-9788821-4-3

Table of Contents

List of Figures

List of Tables

Tables in the Appendices

Acknowledgements

We wish to thank Mark Dinecco and Gianmario Impullitti for their comments on a previous draft, and Chiara Bonassi, Laura Magazzini, Gianluca Papa, Marzia Romanelli and Nicola C. Salerno for skillful research assistance.

Fabio Pammolli

Massimo Riccaboni

Foreward

Bioscience is a critical innovation driver across many economic sectors and a key bellwether of European, North American and Asian competitiveness in a rapidly globalizing economy. In this volume two leading scholars examine the competitive position and performance of pharmaceutical companies and industries in Europe, North America and Japan, as well as China, India, and other emergent economies.

Industrial Leadership and Innovation: Lessons from Pharmaceuticals is the most comprehensive and up-to-date analysis available of the global pharmaceutical industry. Pammolli and Riccaboni explain the strengths and weaknesses of different national systems of regulation and innovation. They examine the evolution of market size and the competitive position of firms, compare employment and productivity levels, look at innovation trends and the international migration of talent, and examine the globalization strategies of leading companies and nations.

Pammolli and Riccaboni compare U.S. and European innovation systems and trace how China and India are accumulating scientific and technological capabilities in the life sciences and in pharmaceuticals.

The results are sobering for Europe. Although European companies still have a solid overall position in pharmaceuticals and some EU countries are performing well, Europe is lagging behind the U.S. in its ability to generate, organize, and sustain innovation processes in pharmaceuticals and resulting productivity growth. Moreover, European industry risks being displaced in the long run by economies with skilled human capital, low labor costs, and great growth potential in terms of both market size and human capital accumulation. Pammolli and Riccaboni advance a concrete agenda of action so Europe can regain competitiveness in pharmaceuticals, and call for renewed transatlantic dialogue on the political economy of the pharmaceutical industry, on trade policy and protection of intellectual property rights.

As part of our mission to address challenges facing the U.S. and Europe in a globalizing world, and as part of our series on transatlantic economic relations, the Center for Transatlantic Relations is pleased to be able to present this outstanding study. I would like to thank the authors for an impressive contribution to understanding the dynamics of the global pharmaceutical industry, and the challenges and opportunities it presents to the United States and Europe.

Daniel Hamilton
Director
Center for Transatlantic Relations

Chapter I
Executive Summary

Chapter I
Executive Summary

This volume examines the competitive position and performance of pharmaceutical companies and industries in Europe, and compares them to some of the major world economies.[1]

In our analysis, we combine two relevant perspectives:

1. the study of industry dynamics and firm-level strategies by reference to the location of corporate headquarters;

2. the analysis of production, trade, and R&D activities by country, regardless of the origin of the companies in question.

Jointly, these approaches provide a fairly coherent picture of the dynamics and determinants of industrial leadership for countries and firms.

Our findings, which will be discussed at length in the following chapters, can be summarized as follows.

Market Share and Market Size

The U.S. pharmaceutical market is not only by far the largest in the world, it has also grown rapidly since the mid 1990s. The U.S. market is now almost twice the size of the EU-15 market. Moreover, U.S. companies significantly increased their share of total world sales from 34 percent in 1989 to 44 percent in 2003. This was not simply a consequence of the U.S. market growing, since U.S. companies gained market share in Europe and in Japan as well.

Although important, the size of the U.S. market is therefore not the only source of U.S. leadership. However, if it is true that trade openness has increased over time in the context of a globalized market, apparently reducing the importance of the size of internal markets, European countries are suffering from excessive regulatory and administrative fragmentation in pharmaceuticals.

---

[1] This volume updates and expand work undertaken for the Directorate General Enterprise of the European Commission in 2000 by Gambardella, Orsenigo and Pammolli entitled, *Global Competitiveness in Pharmaceuticals: A European Perspective* (GOP, 2000).

Employment and Productivity

Employment in the European pharmaceutical industry is higher than in the U.S., yet U.S. pharmaceutical production outperforms Europe and Japan in terms of value of production and share of total manufacturing. Between 1995 and 2003, U.S. production grew at an average annual rate of 8 percent, as compared to an increase of 6.8 percent for the EU-15.

Labor costs are lower in Europe than in the U.S. and the gap between the two values is increasing. In 1995, labor cost per employee was approximately 10 percent lower in the EU-15 than in the U.S. In 2003, the difference was significantly larger (30 percent).

Europe lags behind the U.S. in pharmaceutical labor productivity. Value added per employee in the U.S. is higher than in Europe, with the exception of Ireland and Sweden. Indeed, the labor productivity gap with the U.S. is much larger in pharmaceuticals than in overall manufacturing. In 2003, labor productivity in the European pharmaceutical industry was 53.5 percent that of the U.S.

Overall productivity growth is lower in Europe. Some European countries have experienced higher labor productivity growth rates than the U.S. (e.g. Ireland, Sweden, Denmark, France, UK, and Belgium between 1995 and 2003). However, empirical investigations reveal that to a considerable extent, in these countries productivity gains stem from increased U.S. foreign direct investment (FDI). On the contrary, in Germany, Italy, Spain, and Greece, the main drivers of productivity growth have been, in different periods, exchange rate depreciation and lower labor costs.

The European pharmaceutical industry is more labor-intensive than its U.S. counterpart. Capital accumulation in the U.S. has occurred at consistently faster rates than in the EU. From 1990 to 2003 the U.S. capital stock, measured in real terms, has almost doubled. At the same time, capital accumulation in Europe increased at a rate of only 1.0 percent per year. As a result, in 2003, capital per employee in the U.S. was 56.5 percent higher than the average value measured for the ten largest EU countries (hereafter EU-10).

Since the mid-1990s, U.S. productivity growth has been driven both by TFP growth and capital accumulation (3.8 and 2.6 percent respectively), while the most relevant component in Europe was total factor productivity growth (5.0 percent in 1996-2003), accounting for 84.7 percent of the productivity growth per employee.

In synthesis, the U.S. is solidly heading toward a production model where both technological progress and capital deepening play a relevant role, whereas Europe is headed towards lower value added activities and lower capital intensity.

Strategies to Globalize and the Impact of Economic Integration

Dissimilarities in business and industrial models account for the different performances of the U.S. and the EU in terms of productivity and patterns of internationalization.

On the one side, foreign direct investment of U.S. companies in Europe flows towards locations with productivity conditions analogous to the ones they have in their home country—high labor productivity, skilled labor force, high capital/labor ratio—while simultaneously taking advantage of cheaper production factors due to favorable tax systems and lower labor costs. On the contrary, European investments in the U.S. are mainly "market seeking" investments and/or "knowledge seeking" investments in R&D, contributing to an increasing concentration of science and technology.

The different patterns of internationalization of EU and U.S. multinationals explain to a good extent the U.S. trade deficit with Europe, which is largely due to the increase in the import of pharmaceutical products from U.S. affiliates based in Europe.

Moreover, the delocalization of U.S. manufacturing in pharmaceuticals has contributed to the positive performances of Ireland, Hungary, Sweden, and the UK: in these countries, subsidiaries of foreign multinationals account for more than 80 percent of the total turnover in pharmaceuticals.

Innovation

Since 2000, the U.S. has consolidated its central role as the leading locus of innovation in pharmaceuticals. U.S. firms hold the majority of the global stock of biopharmaceutical patents. This dominant position continues to expand. Moving from the period 1986-1995 to the period 1996-2005, the share of biopharmaceutical patents held by U.S. inventors has risen by approximately 5 percent (from 64.6 percent to 68.2 percent). As shown by the shares of co-invented patents at the international level, U.S. based firms and institutions play a pivotal role in the global division of innovative labor in pharmaceuticals. U.S. dominance is even more pronounced when looking at patent citations, a proxy of patents quality. Patterns of international migration of skilled human capital confirm such a central role, with a consistent flow of high-skill workers from abroad towards the U.S. As an example, the share of EU-25 inventors is higher than the share of EU-25 institutional assignees. The opposite is true for the U.S.: in other words, there are more European inventors in U.S. labs than vice-versa. The capability of U.S. institutions to attract skilled human capital is an important driver of the productivity of the U.S. system.

The difficulties of Europe to attract skilled workers, and the "brain drain" that is experienced, relate to the quality of working conditions. Better prospects and projects and easier access to leading technologies are frequently cited as reasons behind plans to work abroad. To reverse such a negative trend, Europe must reform its higher education system, injecting competition among universities, reducing bureaucracy, and promoting a transformation of its university system into a meritocracy (See Alesina and Giavazzi, 2006).

China and India are accumulating scientific and technological capabilities in the life sciences and in pharmaceuticals, moving towards a knowledge-intensive development pattern. This process, which is also sustained by the structure of high skill "diaspora networks" centered in the U.S., represents a serious challenge for Europe, which might be displaced in the long run by the Asiatic countries, which can benefit from skilled human capital, low labor costs, and great growth potential in terms of both market size and human capital accumulation.

The internal structure of the U.S. national innovation system is a powerful source of competitive advantage and industrial leadership. In the U.S., the biotech sector plays a vital role establishing a bridge and integrating explorations of new research opportunities with clinical and market development. On the contrary, Europe suffers from a lack of dynamism of young technology-dedicated firms in generating and developing R&D projects.

The biotechnology sector in the U.S. has been sustained by the evolution of the U.S. stock market. The stock market boom of the late 1990s greatly increased the favorable conditions for the flourishing of new biotech start-ups. However, while in Europe the bubble bursting caused a significant blow to biotech share prices, in the U.S. the situation was quite different. There, the fine grained R&D network and the highly competitive price structure constituted the breeding ground for the real beginning of a new industrial sector, capable of continuing its activities well after the bursting of the high tech bubble.

R&D Productivity Slowdown

Despite the exponential growth of public and private R&D expenditures during the last 30 years, since 1996 the rate at which the industry generates new molecular entities has been sharply decreasing. In the short run, this evidence explains most of the downturn of U.S. productivity growth in pharmaceuticals. However, it is worth noting that biopharmaceutical products (recombinant therapeutic proteins, monoclonal antibody-based products used for in vivo medical purposes and nucleic acid-based medicinal products) now represent approximately one in every four new molecular entities coming on the market and this share should increase in the future. Hence, U.S. leadership in the biotech sector raises serious concerns about future EU pharmaceutical competitiveness. As we discuss at length in Chapter IV, this productivity slowdown might be the result of multiple factors:

1. R&D opportunities exhaustion (the "fishing out" effect);

2. The impact of new general purpose research technologies and of genomics;

3. Gestation lags and time to market associated with the length and with the complexities of pharmaceutical R&D;

4. Insufficient market incentives and rewards for innovation.

In the long run, for both Europe and the U.S., industrial productivity, as well as the intensity and direction of pharmaceutical innovation, will be affected by the interplay between technological progress and demand regulation, especially in relation to the effective management of health and pharmaceutical expenditures to encourage innovation and quality while preserving the fiscal sustainability of national health systems.

Competition and Regulation

The market for pharmaceuticals in the U.S. is both more concentrated and more volatile than in Europe. Despite its greater concentration, it is fiercely competitive: product turnover is much more rapid than in the EU and Japan, and competition from generics is strong after patent expiry. The U.S. market is in fact an archetype of a classical scheme of Schumpeterian competition, where innovators gain temporary exclusivity positions, thus stimulating innovation and imitation by competitors that leads to more novel products and a high market turnover. Dynamic competition is less pervasive and less intense in the EU, especially in continental Europe. Evidence discussed in Chapter V of this volume shows that market competition in some European countries is in fact weak, with inefficiencies that are reflected in productivity indicators as well as in other performance indicators.

It is difficult to make straightforward comparisons between pharmaceutical prices in the United States and Europe, due to the complexity of the market-based, decentralized, and competitive U.S. pricing environment. Our analysis indicates that U.S. pharmaceutical prices have been more than double the EU-15 average in the past decade. Branded drugs account for this gap, while the prices of U.S. generic drugs are in line with the EU-15 average. In Europe, markets such as the United Kingdom and Germany display higher prices than countries like France and Italy, which rely upon price regulation systems. U.S. prices of generic drugs are substantially aligned with the EU-15 average, but in many cases they are well below European and Canadian prices for generics. More extensive prescribing and use of relatively less expensive generics in the United States has fostered a competitive generics market there, and has helped to free up financial resources that are used in turn to fund greater consumption of innovative drugs by patients for whom those medicines constitute the most appropriate and beneficial treatment option. By artificially constraining prices of innovative medicines in the early stages of product life cycles, while failing to stimulate a robust and competitive market for generic medicines (with notable exceptions like the UK and Germany), European governments are missing an opportunity to create "headroom" for innovation, increasing value for patients and incentives to innovate.

Europe has Strengths but is Lagging: The Way Forward

Europe still has a solid position in pharmaceuticals, and some EU countries are performing well. Europe has a strong trade surplus, including a surplus with the U.S. It is attracting U.S. FDI, and not simply to serve the EU market. It has six of the top 20 pharmaceutical companies. Although U.S. multinationals have performed better overall than European ones in terms of successful new products, the top EU-15 companies in 2005 had a greater proportion of their turnover from new products (launched since 2001) than did U.S. companies. Researchers located in the EU-25 accounted for 25 percent of USPTO granted pharmaceutical patents in the 10 years prior to 2005.

However, Europe is lagging behind the U.S. in pharmaceuticals in terms of market size and production growth, as well as internationalization through market penetration and foreign direct investments. Moreover, over time the European environment has become less attractive for skilled human capital and for the location of R&D activities in biotechnology and pharmaceuticals.

In particular, Europe is lagging behind the U.S. in its ability to generate, organize, and sustain innovation processes in pharmaceuticals. A disproportionate share of pharmaceutical R&D is performed in the U.S., with negative consequences for the EU in terms of both high value-added employment and complementary investments in medical research.

A More Dynamic European Business Climate

According to the evidence presented in this volume, the shortcomings in European competitiveness in pharmaceuticals seem to be induced, among other factors, by the excessive fragmentation of the European environment in: a) research, with the dominance of national systems of innovation; b) market regulation, with high administration and transaction costs preventing the emergence of a single market for pharmaceuticals; c) structure of health care financing, with the dominance of tax based funding schemes defined and implemented at the national level by member states.

The EU pharmaceuticals market suffers at the supranational level from the sort of institutional fragmentation that hindered transactions and stifled economic growth for centuries within European states themselves (Epstein, 2000).

During the 18th and 19th centuries, problems of institutional fragmentation within European states were solved through the establishment of uniform national laws by central governments (see Dincecco, 2006).

We may envision a similar institutional solution with respect to 21st century pharmaceuticals in the European Union. By enabling the EU Commission to enact a uniform set of enforceable legal reforms across countries, such costs would be reduced, making the European pharmaceutical industry more efficient and promoting competition, specialization, and trade.

This is not to suggest, however, that what the European pharmaceutical industry needs for success is greater government involvement, only this time at the supranational level rather than that of individual countries. The free market forces which ultimately drive innovation and competitiveness, rather than the visible hand of the government, should be encouraged. It is to say, however, that the EU Commission requires greater control over the underlying "rules of the game" to establish the sort of legal regime that make for a more competitive, dynamic environment.

The disappointing performance of the European pharmaceutical industry cannot be fully explained by sector-specific factors. It is also the consequence of Europe's relative lack of dynamism in introducing vast institutional changes aimed at improving the overall business environment as well as reforming its labor and capital markets, education systems, public spending, and regimes of market regulation (Alesina and Giavazzi, 2006).

This evidence is not simply the result of patterns of comparative advantage among nations. Especially in knowledge-intensive sectors comparative advantages are "induced" or endogenous, and depend heavily on institutions and policy (Gomory and Baumol, 2001). The big issue here is an old issue in strategic trade policy, i.e., being competitive in high value added sectors is better for national income (specializing in "computer chips is better than potato chips"; Thurow, 1992).

Only by combining sector-specific actions and broad reforms of economic institutions can Europe generate a competitive and attractive business environment for pharmaceuticals.

In particular, there are a number of specific issues the EU needs to address if Europe is to regain competitiveness in pharmaceuticals.

Investment in Public R&D in the Life Sciences and in Biopharmaceuticals

An important factor behind U.S. industrial leadership is the competitive university system, and the close interplay among universities, public research centers, and companies. The interplay among different institutions has often been supported by public intervention through a variety of governmental agencies (i.e. NSF, NIH, DoD), acting as catalysts of innovation, in particular through "mission oriented" research programs financed through competitive research and procurement schemes (see Stokes, 1996). The size of public funding is much greater. For the period 1996-2002 EU-15 private R&D expenditure was as large as that in the U.S., whereas public expenditure was less than 25 percent of that of the U.S. However, the approach also differs. Whereas public intervention in Europe awards the largest share of financing to structures (being a university or a company), in the U.S. funding is more strictly linked to performance and assigned to individual researchers through a peer-reviewed process.

Reduced Price Regulation

For both Europe and the U.S., industrial productivity, as well as the role and direction of pharmaceutical innovation over the long term, will be affected by the interplay between technological advances and patterns of demand, especially in relation to the effective management of health and pharmaceutical expenditures in order to encourage innovation while preserving equity and the fiscal sustainability of national health systems (see Pammolli and Salerno, 2006).

Transatlantic Dialogue

The uneven geographical distribution of research activities in pharmaceuticals, together with the observed differences in price levels for innovative drugs and in reimbursement schemes between Europe and the U.S., as well as across European countries, call for revival of the transatlantic dialogue on the political economy of the pharmaceutical industry, with particular reference to trade policy and the protection of intellectual property rights.

Such a dialogue is crucial, particularly at a time when both EU and U.S. policymakers are trying to balance the goals of encouraging and rewarding innovation, while controlling its economic implications in health care and pharmaceuticals.

Chapter II
Productivity and Competitiveness

Chapter II

Productivity and Competitiveness

Main Findings

- Although EU employment in the pharmaceutical industry is higher than in the U.S., U.S. production is larger and it is increasing at a higher rate than the EU, and considerably faster than Japan, in both absolute terms and as a share of total manufacturing. In 2003, U.S. pharmaceutical production amounts to 123 billion euros, and the compound annual growth rate over the period 1995-2003 equals 8 percent, 1.4 percentage points more than Europe, and 6 percentage points more than Japan.

- Relevant differences exist across European countries. In Ireland, Belgium, Sweden, the Netherlands and Denmark pharmaceutical production has been growing in absolute terms, reaching a share of total manufacturing which is equal to or above the U.S. level (over the period 1995-2003). Unlike small northern EU countries, slower growth characterizes Italy, France, Germany and UK.

- Europe lags behind the U.S. in terms of labor productivity in pharmaceuticals. On average, labor productivity in the European pharmaceutical industry in 2003 was 53.5 percent of that of the U.S. industry. The value added per employee is higher in the U.S. than in any EU country, with the exception of Ireland and Sweden. Even productivity growth is lower in the E.U. with respect to the U.S., though marked differences exist across EU member states. From 1995 to 2003 Ireland, Sweden, Denmark, France, UK, and Belgium have experienced labor productivity growth rates higher than the U.S.

- The positive productivity trend in the EU-15 is driven by the good performance of France, UK and, above all, of small northern European countries, most notably Belgium, Denmark, Ireland and Sweden. As suggested by the evidence presented in Chapter III, in Europe productivity gains largely stem from the rise of U.S. foreign direct investment.

- The productivity gap between the U.S. and the EU-15 in pharmaceuticals is much larger than in total manufacturing, even though the euro depreciation and globalization forces tend to close the gap. In 2001, EU labor productivity in pharmaceuticals was 60 percent of U.S. levels, compared to 81 percent in manufacturing.

- Labor is less expensive in Europe than in the U.S. In 2003, labor cost per employee was 30 percent lower in the EU-15 than in the U.S. However, for a clear understanding of productivity differentials, wages and labor productivity must be considered simultaneously. Even though the EU-15 remains less cost competitive than the U.S., relative pharmaceutical productivity figures have slightly improved in the period from 1995 to 2003, thanks to some EU-15 labor productivity gains and relative (EU-15 versus U.S.) price improvements.

- Small open countries (most notably Belgium, Ireland and Sweden) managed to keep labor costs under control and to raise productivity levels. As a result, unit labor cost (ULC) is very close to U.S. levels, thus attracting significant flows of foreign investments from the U.S.

- The U.S. is steadily heading toward a production model where progress is spearheaded by both technological progress and capital deepening, whereas European countries are edging towards lower value added activities and lower capital intensity. In addition, European countries respond less to the growth of non-labor inputs. Looking at its decomposition, productivity growth in the U.S. could be explained both by total factor productivity (TFP) growth and capital accumulation (3.8 and 2.6 percent average growth in 1996-2003), while the most important component of the EU aggregate was TFP growth (5.0 percent average growth in 1996-2003), accounting for 84.7 percent of labor productivity growth. Capital accumulation in Europe is still modest (1.0 percent average growth in 1996-2003).

- The slowdown of the U.S. TFP growth in pharmaceuticals recorded from the mid-1990s is mostly due to the downturn of R&D productivity within the industry (see Chapter IV).

- Given its "residual nature," TFP therefore captures not only firms' heterogeneity, but also institutional heterogeneity across countries. Strong competition and deregulation, which are distinctive features of the U.S. institutional setting (see Chapter V), lead firms to increase investments. Hence the effects of competition can unfold through increased capital accumulation as well as through TFP growth.

II.1   Overview

This chapter examines the competitiveness of European pharmaceutical sector *vis-à-vis* the U.S. The analysis relies upon country-level data from the OECD-STAN database to compute labor productivity, unit labor cost, capital accumulation, and Total Factor Productivity (TFP) over the last 20 years.

We compare the pharmaceutical labor productivity and labor cost at the international level and employ traditional growth accounting techniques to measure productivity trends.

GOP (2000) described the European industry as higher labor-intensive, performing lower value added activities, and less responsive to growth in non-labor inputs. Those results are confirmed by the analysis in this chapter.

Moreover, we compare our results for the pharmaceutical industry with those of manufacturing in general, in order to find out whether they are likely determined by sector-specific competitive forces or economy-wide factors. In the EU case, the pharmaceutical industry shows productivity trends partially similar to those of the whole manufacturing sector, suggesting widespread institutional and competitive forces at play. The global trends in GDP per capita and the decomposition of real GDP also highlight the importance of national and regional competitiveness forces. In contrast to the United States, EU institutions, and more generally EU cultural attitudes have been less favorable to the kind of Schumpeterian "creative destruction" that plays a key role in fostering long-term economic growth in all sectors including pharmaceuticals (Phelps 2003; Gordon 2004; Alesina and Giavazzi 2006).

Employment in the pharmaceutical industry is considerably higher in the EU than in the U.S. In 2003, pharmaceutical firms based in the EU-

15 countries employed more than 483,000 workers, equal to 1.8 percent of total employment. The corresponding figures for the U.S. are about 270,000 employees, 1.7 percent share of total employment in 2003.

The U.S. had an average annual growth rate in pharmaceutical employment of 1.6 percent from 1995 to 2003, compared to 1 percent in the EU-15 and 0.1 percent in Japan.

Strong differences emerge among European countries, however. At one extreme, Ireland, Sweden and Belgium have experienced sharp increases in their pharmaceutical labor force, recording annual growth rates of 6.7, 3.8 and 3.7 percent respectively. At another extreme, Greece is the country with the largest decrease over the period 1995-2003 (-3.0 percent). UK employment has been declining during the 1990s too, and even though this trend reversed between 2000 and 2002, reaching a peak up to more than 78,000 workers, it started to decline again in 2003.

Comparing growth rates across the two periods (1990-1995 vs. 1995-2003), we observe an increase of pharmaceutical employment in most European countries. In Austria, Denmark, Sweden, Norway and Ireland positive growth trend have started right at the beginning of the 1990s. In particular, Ireland has experienced the highest growth of the pharmaceutical workforce: the average annual growth rate was more than 9 percent over the period 1990-1995, and 6.7 percent from 1995 to 2003. On the contrary, pharmaceutical employment decreased in France, Germany, Italy, Spain, the UK and the Netherlands over the first half of the 1990s. However, in some of these countries (France, Germany, Italy and the Netherlands), employment started to grow again in 1995-2003, even if only in the cases of Germany and the Netherlands the total headcount was higher in 2003 than in 1990.

Although employment in the European pharmaceutical industry is higher than in the U.S., U.S. pharmaceutical production is more or less the same as in Europe (see Table II.2). Between 1995 and 2003, U.S. production grew at an average annual rate of 8 percent, a little faster than the EU-15 (growth rate of 6.8 percent) and considerably faster than Japan (growth rate of 2 percent). However, it has to be noted that the value of U.S. pharmaceutical production has been declining since 2001 in nominal terms, due to dollar depreciation, while it is increasing in real terms.

Table II.1 Number of employees in pharmaceuticals as a share of total manufacturing employment (*in italics*)

Countries	1990	1995	2000	2001	2002	2003	Average[1] '90-'95	Average[1] '95-'03
EU-15[2]	—	451,017	470,014	471,730	492,187*	488,435*	—	1.0%
	—	*1.5%*	*1.6%*	*1.7%*	*1.8%*	*1.8%*	—	*0.03%*
U.S.	206,046	238,623	268,606	276,224	270,513	270,119	3.0%	1.6%
	1.1%	*1.3%*	*1.4%*	*1.5%*	*1.6%*	*1.7%*	*0.04%*	*0.05%*
Japan	120,687	117,500	123,169	123,126	120,045	117,975	-0.5%	0.1%
	0.8%	*0.9%*	*1.0%*	*1.0%*	*1.0%*	*1.0%*	*0.01%*	*0.02%*
Germany	121,107	113,294	120,120	120,574	121,537*	130,467*	-1.3%	1.8%
	1.2%	*1.3%*	*1.5%*	*1.5%*	*1.5%*	*1.7%*	*0.04%*	*0.04%*
Italy	87,131	73,131	82,780	80,036	81,838	81,930*	-3.4%	1.4%
	1.6%	*1.4%*	*1.6%*	*1.6%*	*1.6%*	*1.6%*	*-0.03%*	*0.02%*
France	71,300	70,700	68,800	71,600	73,900	71,342*	-0.2%	0.1%
	1.6%	*1.8%*	*1.8%*	*1.9%*	*2.0%*	*1.9%*	*0.04%*	*0.01%*
UK	73,948	70,033	63,302	64,663	78,369	67,722*	-1.1%	-0.4%
	1.4%	*1.6%*	*1.5%*	*1.6%*	*2.0%*	*1.8%*	*0.03%*	*0.03%*
Spain	42,063	40,049	39,521	43,019	40,420	42,292*	-1.0%	0.7%
	1.5%	*1.6%*	*1.4%*	*1.5%*	*1.4%*	*1.5%*	*0.02%*	*-0.02%*
Canada	23,463	23,336	27,677	28,862	27,011	28,877	-0.1%	2.7%
	1.1%	*1.2%*	*1.3%*	*1.3%*	*1.3%*	*1.3%*	*0.02%*	*0.01%*
Poland[3]	—	25,671	26,006	25,101	26,331*	25,320*	—	-0.2%
	—	*0.8%*	*1.0%*	*1.0%*	*1.0%*	*1.0%*	—	*0.02%*
Belgium	—	15,539	18,166	19,078	20,063*	20,772*	—	3.7%
	—	*2.3%*	*2.8%*	*2.9%*	*3.2%*	*3.4%*	—	*0.14%*
Sweden	13,909	14,473	17,434	18,858	19,942	19,523*	0.8%	3.8%
	1.6%	*1.9%*	*2.3%*	*2.5%*	*2.7%*	*2.7%*	*0.07%*	*0.09%*
Netherlands	14,940	14,508	16,209	16,243	17,352	16,014*	-0.6%	1.2%
	1.3%	*1.4%*	*1.5%*	*1.5%*	*1.6%*	*1.6%*	*0.01%*	*0.03%*
Denmark	10,758	11,955	12,805	13,045	13,162	13,368	2.1%	1.4%
	2.1%	*2.5%*	*2.8%*	*2.9%*	*3.0%*	*3.2%*	*0.08%*	*0.08%*
Ireland	4,225	6,593	10,094	10,972	11,786	11,037*	9.3%	6.7%
	1.9%	*2.6%*	*3.4%*	*3.6%*	*4.1%*	*3.9%*	*0.2%*	*0.2%*
Austria	8,937	9,453	10,454	9,337	9,575	9,811*	1.1%	0.5%
	1.2%	*1.4%*	*1.6%*	*1.4%*	*1.5%*	*1.5%*	*0.04%*	*0.02%*
Greece	—	7,113	6,124	—	—	—	—	-3.0%
	—	*1.1%*	*1.0%*	—	—	—	—	*-0.02%*
Finland	4,067	4,175	4,206	4,306	4,243*	3,960*	0.5%	-0.7%
	0.8%	*1.0%*	*0.9%*	*0.9%*	*0.9%*	*0.9%*	*0.04%*	*-0.01%*
Norway	2,200	3,100	3,600	3,600	3,700	3,818*	7.1%	2.6%
	0.7%	*1.0%*	*1.2%*	*1.2%*	*1.3%*	*1.4%*	*0.06%*	*0.05%*

(1) Compound Annual Growth Rate (absolute figures); annual average change (percentage figures in italics). (2) Does not include Portugal for the whole period and Greece in 2001. (3) 1996 instead of 1995. (*)Projections based on Eurostat survey data.

Source: OECD-STAN

Table II.2   Total production of pharmaceuticals in current € millions and as a share of total manufacturing production (*in italics*)

Countries	1990	1995	2000	2001	2002	2003	Average[1] '90-'95	Average[1] '95-'03
U.S.	43,779	60,750	125,338	141,156	133,977	123,121	7.3%	8.0%
	1.9%	*2.2%*	*2.6%*	*3.0%*	*3.1%*	*3.3%*	*0.06%*	*0.14%*
EU-15[2]	—	88,251	126,891	135,313	145,705*	149,094*	—	6.8%
	—	*2.4%*	*2.6%*	*2.8%*	*3.0%*	*3.1%*	—	*0.09%*
Japan	33,981	54,832	72,529	70,068	64,261	60,498	1.5%	2.0%
	1.9%	*2.2%*	*2.4%*	*2.6%*	*2.8%*	*2.8%*	*0.06%*	*0.08%*
France	15,699	21,721	27,707	30,508	31,763	32,776*	5.4%	5.4%
	2.8%	*3.4%*	*3.5%*	*3.7%*	*3.9%*	*3.5%*	*0.1%*	*0.05%*
Germany	12,974	18,035	22,893	24,304	24,760*	27,929*	4.7%	6.2%
	1.4%	*1.7%*	*1.8%*	*1.9%*	*1.9%*	*2.2%*	*0.04%*	*0.03%*
UK	8,739	12,189	19,144	20,822	22,382	20,667	10.0%	4.4%
	2.1%	*2.6%*	*2.8%*	*3.1%*	*3.5%*	*3.5%*	*0.1%*	*0.08%*
Italy	15,770	12,210	17,747	18,090	21,298	19,566*	1.5%	4.8%
	2.7%	*2.2%*	*2.4%*	*2.4%*	*2.8%*	*2.6%*	*-0.1%*	*0.04%*
Korea	4,708	8,943	12,311	11,740	12,568	10,977	16.3%	6.3%
	2.2%	*2.3%*	*2.1%*	*2.1%*	*2.2%*	*2.1%*	*0.03%*	*-0.03%*
Spain	5,305	6,263	7,981	9,126	9,219	9,911*	8.3%	6.2%
	2.3%	*2.4%*	*2.2%*	*2.4%*	*2.4%*	*2.5%*	*0.01%*	*0.02%*
Belgium	1,880	3,668	6,212	7,398	8,053*	8,880*	12.0%	12.3%
	1.6%	*2.6%*	*3.5%*	*4.1%*	*4.7%*	*5.2%*	*0.2%*	*0.3%*
Canada	2,679	2,885	5,435	6,536	—	—	5.3%	9.8%
	1.3%	*1.2%*	*1.2%*	*1.5%*	—	—	*-0.01%*	*0.04%*
Netherlands	1,988	3,575	6,214	6,505	7,366	7,387*	10.2%	10.1%
	1.5%	*2.1%*	*2.9%*	*3.1%*	*3.5%*	*3.5%*	*0.1%*	*0.2%*
Sweden	1,898	3,411	5,726	5,963	6,870	7,757*	17.3%	10.5%
	1.7%	*3.0%*	*3.4%*	*3.8%*	*4.5%*	*4.7%*	*0.3%*	*0.1%*
Ireland	626	1,736	4,821	5,028	5,885	5,750*	23.9%	15.7%
	2.4%	*4.2%*	*5.1%*	*5.1%*	*5.9%*	*5.8%*	*0.4%*	*0.2%*
Denmark	1,068	1,923	3,746	3,873	4,032	4050	10.8%	9.9%
	2.3%	*3.3%*	*5.4%*	*5.4%*	*5.5%*	*5.6%*	*0.2%*	*0.4%*
Australia[3]	1,327	2,185	3,250	—	—	—	12.3%	8.6%
	1.3%	*1.9%*	*2.3%*	—	—	—	*0.1%*	*0.1%*
Austria	1,177	1,728	2,572	1,988	2,252	2,465*	5.8%	5.1%
	1.7%	*2.0%*	*2.4%*	*1.8%*	*2.0%*	*2.2%*	*0.06%*	*-0.03%*
Poland[4]	—	937	1,165	1,538	1,618*	1,572*	—	11.50%
	—	*1.3%*	*1.1%*	*1.3%*	*1.4%*	*1.4%*	—	*0.02%*
Hungary	—	700	1,024	1,223	1,308	1,585*	7.5%	16.8%
	—	*3.2%*	*2.1%*	*2.3%*	*2.4%*	*2.7%*	*0.6%*	*-0.2%*
Portugal	584	781	1,045	998	1,125*	1,082*	7.7%	4.4%
	1.3%	*1.5%*	*1.6%*	*1.5%*	*1.7%*	*1.6%*	*0.03%*	*-0.01%*

Table II.2 *continued*

Countries	1990	1995	2000	2001	2002	2003	Average[1] '90-'95	Average[1] '95-'03
Norway	347	529	1,085	985	1,094	1,044*	9.7%	8.3%
	0.9%	*1.2%*	*1.8%*	*1.6%*	*1.7%*	*1.8%*	*0.1%*	*0.1%*
Finland	451	468	611	710	699*	685*	4.0%	5.5%
	0.7%	*0.7%*	*0.6%*	*0.7%*	*0.7%*	*0.7%*	*-0.01%*	*0.0%*
Greece	—	543	473	—	—	—	-0.8%	—
	—	*1.6%*	*1.1%*	—	—	—	*-0.1%*	—

(1) Compound Annual Growth Rate (values in national currencies, euros used for the EU aggregate); annual average change for percentage values in italics. (2) Does not include Greece in 2001. (3) 1999 instead of 2000. (4) 1996 instead of 1995. (*) Projections based on Eurostat survey data.

Source: OECD-STAN

In 2004, the pharmaceutical industry was the fourth largest three-digit manufacturing sub-sector by production in the U.S. (3.7 percent of total production) and the sixth in the EU-25 (three percent of total production).

However, significant differences exist among European countries in terms of share of production in total manufacturing, ranging from 0.7 percent in Finland to almost six percent in Ireland.

With the sole exception of Finland, where a weak regime of property rights has undermined the growth of a competitive domestic industry, northern European countries are those where the importance of the pharmaceutical sector in total production is substantial. Denmark was the second country, after Ireland, with the highest share in 2003 (5.6 percent). Sweden also displays a high pharmaceutical share of total manufacturing, equal to 4.5 percent.

In terms of growth, over the period 1995-2003, the Netherlands, Ireland, Sweden, Belgium, and Denmark outperformed the U.S. As far as production growth is concerned, the average annual growth rates of pharmaceutical production over the period 1995-2003 ranged from 15.7 percent in Ireland to -0.8 percent in Greece, which has also experienced a decrease in the share of pharmaceutical on total manufacturing (-0.1 percent). In comparison with the first half of the 1990s, in most European countries the growth rate of production decreased, particularly in the UK, whose growth rate declined from 10 percent in 1990-1995 to 4.4 percent in 1995-2003, and in Sweden (from 17.3 percent in 1990-1995 to 10.5 percent in 1995-2003).

The United States outperformed the European Union and Japan, also in terms of value added. Value added is defined as the value of production less costs of intermediate inputs. Therefore, it measures the contribution of the internal factors of production, mainly labor and capital. In 2004, the pharmaceutical industry was the largest 3-digit manufacturing sub-sector in the U.S. economy in terms of value added and the fourth largest in the EU-25.

In 2004, the drug industry in the U.S. accounted for more than 5.9 percent of total manufacturing value added, while its share was far lower in the EU, being equal to 3.7 percent. However, there is an increase over time across countries, both in absolute and in relative terms. By comparing the two sub-periods 1990-1995 and 1995-2003, it is straightforward to note that in the U.S. and the EU the average annual growth rates of the pharmaceutical value added have been accelerating. On the contrary, the Japanese growth rate has sharply declined, from 10 percent to less than one percent.

Germany, France, UK and Italy account for more than 65 percent of the European drug industry's value added. From 1990 to 2003, all these countries increased the share of pharmaceuticals in total manufacturing, though without reaching the level of Sweden (9.3 percent), Ireland (8.5 percent) and Denmark (8.5 percent).

In recent years Italy has experienced a particularly high dynamism, with an average annual growth rate in pharmaceuticals of eight percent and a share of total manufacturing of 4.5 percent, reversing the negative trends of the first half of the 1990s. The opposite holds for France and Germany, while pharmaceuticals in the UK have contributed to a larger extent to the national value added, with growth of pharmaceutical value added of 6.9 percent compound annual growth rate for the period 1995-2003. In 1995-2003, value added in pharmaceutical for Ireland, Sweden, Denmark and Belgium increased at a lower rate than in the previous years, even though its share over manufacturing is steadily high.

In sum, beginning in the second half of the 1990s, the U.S. value added has surpassed that of the EU-15 despite dollar depreciation, with comparable levels of production and almost half the number of EU-15 employees.

Table II.3   Value added of pharmaceuticals in current € millions as a share of total manufacturing value added (*in italics*)

Countries	1990	1995	2000	2001	2002	2003	CAGR[1] '90-'95	CAGR[1] '95-'03
EU-15[2]	26,903	34,849	49,270	54,127	55,641	58,069	5.3%	6.6%
	2.5%	*2.8%*	*3.3%*	*3.5%*	*3.6%*	*3.8%*	*2.3%*	*3.9%*
U.S.	19,206	29,024	59,578	71,036	70,945	68,132	8.6%	11.3%
	3.1%	*3.2%*	*3.6%*	*3.6%*	*4.3%*	*4.5%*	*0.5%*	*4.3%*
Japan[5]	17.000	27.000	34.000	32.000	30.000	28.000	10.0%	0.8%
	2.6%	*2.9%*	*3.0%*	*3.4%*	*3.5%*	*3.6%*	*2.2%*	*2.7%*
Germany	5,659	7,996	8,930	9,993	9,805	11,194	7.2%	4.3%
	1.7%	*2.0%*	*1.8%*	*1.9%*	*2.3%*	*2.6%*	*3.3%*	*3.1%*
Italy	5,688	4,413	7,230	7,838	8,066	8,149	-4.9%	8.0%
	2.9%	*2.5%*	*3.3%*	*3.5%*	*3.3%*	*3.5%*	*-2.9%*	*4.5%*
France	4,587	7,122	9,053	10,099	10,260	10,986	9.2%	5.6%
	2.5%	*3.5%*	*3.8%*	*4.1%*	*4.1%*	*4.5%*	*7.0%*	*3.3%*
UK	4,606	5,308	8,895	10,311	9,958	9,068	2.9%	6.9%
	2.8%	*3.1%*	*3.6%*	*4.2%*	*4.3%*	*4.3%*	*2.1%*	*4.2%*
Spain	2,231	2,264	2,591	3,062	2,935	3,076	0.3%	3.9%
	2.7%	*2.8%*	*2.5%*	*2.9%*	*2.7%*	*2.7%*	*0.7%*	*-0.3%*
Canada	1,482	1,348	1,905	2,486	—	—	-1.9%	—
	2.1%	*1.8%*	*1.3%*	*1.8%*	—	—	*-3.0%*	—
Poland[3]	—	386	567	1,036	841	—	—	—
	—	*1.8%*	*1.60%*	—	—	—	—	—
Portugal	151	300	333	314	341*	346*	14.7%	1.8%
	1.5%	*2.0%*	*1.8%*	*1.6%*	*1.7%*	*1.8%*	*5.9%*	*-1.3%*
Belgium	930	1,722	2,563	2,952	3,174	3,379	13.1%	8.8%
	2.9%	*4.3%*	*5.8%*	*6.8%*	*7.3%*	*7.8%*	*8.2%*	*7.7%*
Sweden	928	1,722	3,002	3,198	3,878	4,400	13.1%	12.4%
	2.6%	*4.5%*	*5.9%*	*7.0%*	*8.4%*	*9.3%*	*11.6%*	*9.5%*
Netherlands	544	1,257	1,547	1,525	1,249	1,184	18.2%	-0.7%
	1.3%	*2.4%*	*2.6%*	*2.5%*	*2.1%*	*2.0%*	*13.0%*	*-2.5%*
Denmark	573	1,008	1,799	1,877	2,086	2,159	12.0%	10.0%
	3.5%	*4.8%*	*7.4%*	*7.6%*	*8.3%*	*8.5%*	*6.5%*	*7.4%*
Ireland	290	882	2,316	2,299	3,140	3,168	24.9%	17.3%
	3.3%	*6.4%*	*7.8%*	*7.0%*	*8.5%*	*8.5%*	*14.2%*	*3.6%*
Austria	480	752	942	660	811	1,017	9.4%	3.9%
	2.0%	*2.4%*	*2.5%*	*1.7%*	*2.0%*	*2.5%*	*3.7%*	*0.6%*
Greece	127	157	139	—	—	—	4.4%	—
	1.3%	*1.5%*	*1.0%*	—	—	—	*2.9%*	—
Finland	260	248	265	312	278	290	-1.0%	2.0%
	7.2%	*6.8%*	*6.3%*	*7.1%*	*6.3%*	*6.6%*	*-1.1%*	*-0.4%*
Norway	151	262	357	368	434	407	11.6%	5.7%
	1.4%	*2.0%*	*2.0%*	*2.0%*	*2.2%*	*2.4%*	*7.4%*	*2.3%*

(1) Compound Annual Growth Rate (national currencies, euros used for EU aggregate); annual average change for percentage values in italics. (2) Does not include Greece in 2001. (3) 1999 instead of 2000. (4) 1996 instead of 1995. (*) Projections based on Eurostat survey data.

Source: OECD-STAN

II.2   International Comparison of Labor Productivity

In this section we analyze cross-country labor productivity gains relying on value added statistics in order to capture the net contribution of pharmaceuticals to economic growth.

Table II.4 shows data on pharmaceutical labor productivity (value-added per employee, in 1997-PPP thousand U.S. dollars) for the period 1980-2003, together with average annual growth rates. Europe lags behind the U.S. as far as pharmaceutical labor productivity is concerned. By comparing sector specific performances with total manufacturing, we find that U.S. productivity leadership holds in general, even though the productivity gap with the U.S. is much larger in pharmaceuticals than in other manufacturing sectors (Figure II.1).[1] Over time, the productivity differential has been reduced, but the competitive advantage of the U.S. in pharmaceuticals has remained unchanged. Few countries, i.e. Ireland and Sweden, are exceptions to this general tendency, displaying levels of value added per employee higher than that of the U.S.

In 2003, EU-15 labor productivity was 53.5 percent that of the U.S. Moreover, recent data reveal an increase in U.S. productivity growth (6.4 percent versus 5.8 percent in the EU-15), widening the gap.

Also in terms of growth, the overall increase in productivity in EU-15 is lower than in the U.S. However, there are some differences within Europe. From 1996 to 2003, the best performers in terms of labor productivity growth rates have been Ireland (9.1), Sweden (9.1), Denmark (8.4), France (7.4), UK (6.8), and Belgium (6.8), each of them have experienced a labor productivity growth rate higher than that of the U.S. In particular, Ireland and Sweden have reached the highest productivity levels among EU countries. However, their con-

---

[1] One of the factors behind the output differentials per worker between Europe and the U.S. is the different amount of hours worked. In general, since the 1970s Europe has experienced a decline, while in the U.S. the total hours worked per worker have risen. Part of the literature (see, Blanchard, 2004) states that this is mainly the outcome of the process of substitution of leisure for income occurring in Europe, a matter of voluntary choice over a different set of preferences between European and American workers, as productivity increases (measuring productivity as output per hour worked, instead of output per worker). However, there is also a less "optimistic" point of view (see, De la Dehesa, 2006, and Alesina-Giavazzi, 2006): the choice made by the European workers is the result of increasing distortions, such as higher taxes on work (see, Prescott, 2004), higher minimum wages, generous or forced early retirement programs.

tribution to aggregate EU productivity is low, due to their relatively small size. Interestingly, much of the productivity increase in these two countries is accounted for by local affiliates of foreign multinational companies.[2]

This evidence, coupled with well-established empirical findings that foreign-owned subsidiaries are more productive than local firms,[3] suggests that the good performances of northern European countries are led by the presence of foreign, mostly U.S., multinational companies (see results in Chapter III).

On the other side, overall EU-15 performance is driven downward by low productivity in Greece, Spain, Finland, Italy and Germany. In particular, the last two countries, with their low productivity levels and high share of EU pharmaceutical value added (a third of the total) negatively affect overall EU-15 productivity in pharmaceuticals (see Table II.4).

Among the new EU member states we observe different country-specific dynamics. On the one hand, in the last few years Hungary has increased its labor productivity at double digits rates (20 percent), gaining a competitive advantage with respect to Germany and Italy. On the other hand, the Czech Republic is still lagging behind, notwithstanding increased productivity in pharmaceuticals, while Poland, for the available years, displays a decreasing productivity trend.

The analysis of the relationship between labor productivity in pharmaceuticals and the share of pharmaceuticals over total manufacturing in Figure II.2 shows that countries' pharmaceutical competitiveness leads to higher specialization in the drug industry. This relationship is particularly strong for Ireland and Denmark, while it is weaker for other top performers such as Japan and the U.S. suggesting the prevalence of sector-specific factors in the former cases and wider institutional (non-industry specific) sources of competitive advantage in the latter.

---

[2] In Ireland, between 70 percent and 80 percent of value added in the manufacturing sector was generated by firms under foreign control. In France, Sweden and the Netherlands this ratio was between 25 percent and 30 percent. In other countries, it was below 20 percent. Labor productivity (value added per employee) of foreign affiliates in the manufacturing sector was greater than the national average in all countries for which data are available (OECD, 2005).

[3] Djankov and Murrell (2002) provide an interesting survey of the literature on this issue. See also, Blomstrom (1986) and Aitken and Harrison (1999).

Purchasing Power Parity (PPP) and International Productivity Comparison

In order to compare productivity levels over time, we need to net out fluctuations in prices and exchange rates. Currency conversion at a reference year (USD in 1997[1]) is based on the methodology developed by the GGDC Group at the University of Groningen for the International Comparisons of Output and Productivity (hereafter "ICOP"). The ICOP programme aims at defining sectoral purchasing power parities (hereafter "PPPs"), to better compare productivities of industrial and services sectors between countries and over time.

These sectoral PPPs are better than whole GDP-PPPs since they take into account the sometimes large sectoral variations in relative prices and therefore have to be preferred to avoid serious distortions. In order to calculate these PPPs, authors compare the relative prices of a representative sample of products for each sector present in both countries.

Since the sectoral level of detail taken into consideration by this program is not sufficient to include the pharmaceutical sector, we use instead chemical sector PPPs and deflators obtained by the GGDC group.

The methodology consists of two steps:

1. First, we use the sectoral deflator (hereafter "DEFL") for each country, in order to express the nominal value of production in constant 1997 prices in national currency;

2. Second, we use the sectoral PPP in order to obtain the real value of production netting out the international differentials of sectoral price levels in 1997.

The first step is to remove the increase in production value due to sectoral price inflation. In the second step we take away from labor productivity the international differentials of sectoral price levels in 1997.

In formulas:

$$\mathrm{LP}_{EU}^{\$97} = \mathrm{LP}_{EU}^{€cy}\,\mathrm{DEFL}^{€97/€cy}/\mathrm{PPP}^{€97/\$97}\,,$$

where:

$\mathrm{LP}_{EU}^{\$97}$ = labor productivity of EU-15 expressed in USD 1997 PPP;

$\mathrm{LP}_{EU}^{€cy}$ = labor productivity of EU-15 expressed in Euros current year;

$\mathrm{DEFL}^{€97/€cy}$ = sectoral deflator between current year and 1997;
$\mathrm{PPP}^{€97/\$97}$ = sectoral purchasing power parity factor EU-15/ U.S. in 1997.

---

[1] Year 1997 has been chosen to use sectoral PPP from the Groningen Growth and Development Centre (60-Industry database).

Figure II.1 Labor productivity, EU vs. U.S., manufacturing and pharmaceuticals, 1980-2001 (U.S.=100)

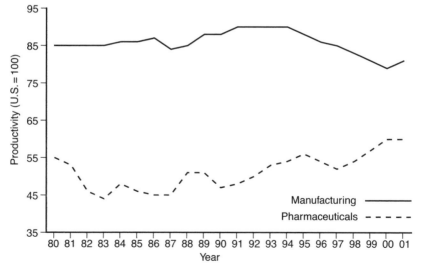

European pharmaceutical productivity has been calculated for the aggregate EU-8 which includes: Austria, Germany, Denmark, Finland, France, UK, Italy and Sweden.

Source: our computations on OECD-STAN, OECD—Main Economic Indicators and GGDC 60-industry database (for pharmaceuticals); GGDC ICOP Database 1997 Benchmark (for manufacturing)

Table II.4 Real value added per employee in the pharmaceutical industry—labor productivity (1997-PPP € thousands)

Country	Value Added						2003 (U.S. =100)	Annual Growth			
	1980	1985	1990	1995	2001	2003[1]		'80-'85	'85-'90	'90-'95	'95-'03
Austria	26.2	29.0	48.9	66.8	64.2	93.5	41.3	2.0%	10.5%	6.2%	4.2%
Belgium	—	—	—	100.2	162.6	172.4	76.1	—	—	—	6.8%
Germany	33.9	37.3	42.1	59.2	78.0	81.3	35.9	1.9%	2.4%	6.8%	4.0%
Denmark	42.4	43.5	47.2	71.1	144.9	138.7	61.3	0.5%	1.6%	8.2%	8.4%
Spain	42.0	41.9	59.0	70.6	80.6	78.6	34.7	0.0%	6.8%	3.6%	1.3%
Finland	46.8	52.8	52.0	51.2	67.0	72.0	31.8	2.4%	-0.3%	-0.3%	4.2%
France	26.8	42.0	65.6	95.3	148.3	172.1	76.0	9.0%	8.9%	7.5%	7.4%
UK	34.8	43.1	60.8	77.9	141.0	133.8	59.1	4.3%	6.9%	5.0%	6.8%
Greece[2]	—	—	—	19.3	20.5	—	—	—	—	—	—
Ireland	—	—	61.1	115.6	155.4	239.0	105.6	—	—	12.8%	9.1%
Italy	36.2	58.8	71.9	73.5	97.2	99.2	43.8	9.7%	4.0%	0.4%	3.7%
Netherlands[3]	—	54.2	45.8	85.4	118.1	107.0	47.3	—	-5.6%	12.5%	2.8%
Portugal[4]	—	—	—	37.9	58.5	67.6	29.9	—	—	—	8.3%
Sweden	35.2	46.5	62.0	116.1	173.8	241.0	106.5	5.6%	5.8%	12.5%	9.1%
EU-8[5]	33.5	44.2	57.7	75.3	112.4	120.2	53.1	5.5%	5.3%	5.3%	5.8%
EU-15[6]	—	—	—	76.7	112.7	121.0	53.5	—	—	—	5.7%
U.S.	61.4	96.2	121.9	135.3	186.1	226.4	100.0	9.0%	4.7%	2.1%	6.4%
Japan	35.0	76.6	113.3	133.6	159.6	183.6	81.1	15.6%	7.8%	3.3%	4.0%
Czech Rep.[7]	—	—	—	—	47.6	54.9	24.3	—	—	—	4.8%
Hungary[8]	—	—	—	52.6	104.0	144.6	63.9	—	—	—	20.2%
Poland[9]	—	—	—	52.5	28.4	—	—	—	—	—	—
Canada	22.7	47.4	63.8	83.2	84.2	—	—	—	14.7%	5.9%	5.3%	—
Norway	33.6	44.0	79.1	69.8	55.6	—	—	—	5.4%	11.7%	-2.5%	—

(1)Projections based on Eurostat survey data (except for Denmark and the U.S.). (2) 2000 instead of 2001. (3) 1987-1990 instead of 1986-1990. (4) The EU-8 aggregate includes: Austria, Germany, Denmark, Finland, France, UK, Italy and Sweden. (5) Excluding Greece, Luxembourg and Portugal. (7) Period 2000-2003. (8) Period 1998-2003. (9) Period 1996-2001.

Source: our computations on OECD-STAN, OECD—Main Economic Indicators, Eurostat and GGDC (latest data available)

Figure II.2   Relative labor productivity versus share of pharmaceuticals over manufacturing, 2001

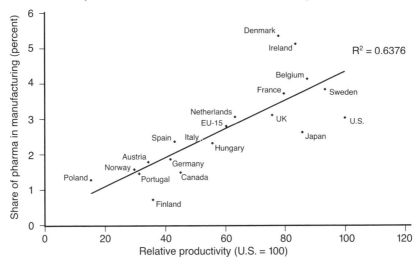

Source: our computations on OECD-STAN

II.3   Pharmaceutical Cost Competitiveness

In the previous section we have witnessed that, overall, higher labor productivity provides U.S. pharmaceutical firms with important competitive advantages over those in Europe and Japan, albeit some differences emerge across Europe. Against this background, in this section we ponder productivity differentials with cost competitiveness.

Table II.5 reports the labor cost per employee and its average growth rate. Clearly, labor is less expensive in Europe than in the U.S. and the cost advantage of Europe has grown larger in the last few years. In 1995, labor cost per employee was approximately 10 percent lower in EU-15 than in the U.S. In 2003, this gap was three times wider.

The euro-dollar exchange rate swing mostly explains the dynamics of EU cost competitiveness. Indeed, the double-digit growth rates in 1986-1990 and lower growth rates both in 1981-1985 and 1996-2001 closely reflect the effects of two episodes of sharp appreciation of the U.S. dollar, culminating in 1985 (with subsequent sharp depreciation) and in 2001 (Figure II.3). The relative evolution of labor cost per employee in total manufacturing *vis-à-vis* the U.S. also supports this

Figure II.3   Annual Real Effective Exchange Rates (REER) of the U.S. and EU-15 against the rest of IC24 group (1999 = 100). Nominal unit labor cost deflator, total economy

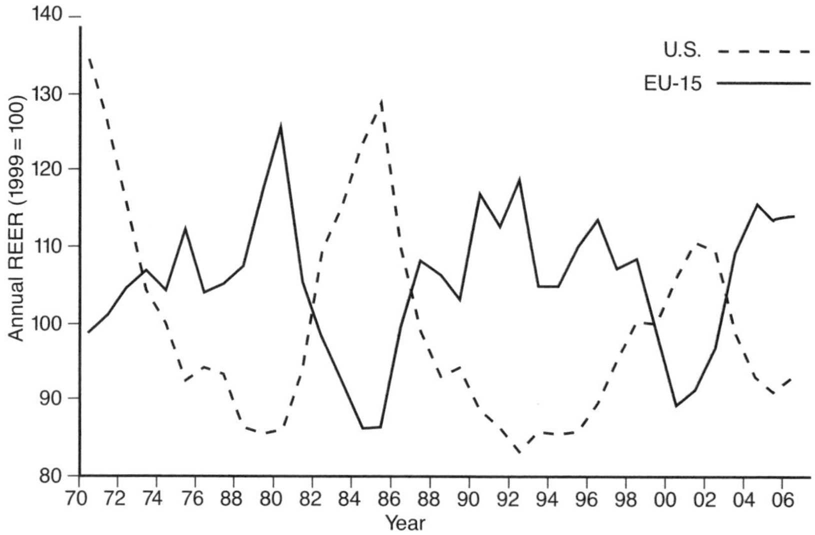

Source: EU Commission (2006a)

view, as labor compensation in pharmaceuticals closely follows fluctuations in aggregate manufacturing (Figure II.4).

As for labor productivity, there is a considerable variation inside the EU aggregate. On the one hand, Greece, Ireland and Finland have the lowest labor costs per employee, while, on the other hand, the UK displays the highest, close to that of the U.S. Also in terms of growth rate, the UK follows the U.S. trend, with an increase of labor costs higher than 8 percent from 1996 to 2003. Even Denmark and Italy have experienced high growth rates, while Austria is the European country showing the most stable pattern, with an increase of only 0.8 percent.

New EU member states display a common pattern characterized by considerably lower labor costs and double-digit growth rates since late 1991, when most of the price liberalization measures have been completed. This evidence reflects the departure from the compressed wage structure in place during the communist regime toward the EU labor market settings. By and large in all these countries throughout the process of catching up the rate of protection afforded by the real effective exchange rate to domestic companies and foreign affiliates has been rapidly eroded by high rates of inflation and insufficient growth in productivity (Drabek and Brada, 1998; Begg 1998). Up to now eastern European countries have benefited from a competitive advantage with respect to other industrialized economies in terms of lower labor cost, allowing them to be large recipients of foreign investments that in turn have fostered their economic growth. However, unless productivity gains offset the loss of cost competitiveness, emerging countries like China, India, Turkey and others with lower labor cost and higher productivity growth can threaten the ability of the new EU member states to retain a competitive edge on the international markets.[5]

The case of eastern Europe clarifies why to get a comprehensive view of productivity differentials across countries, compensation of employees and labor productivity have to be considered at once. A commonly used measure to assess cost competitiveness is Unit Labor Cost (hereafter "ULC").

For the period 1980-2003, Figure II.5 shows the evolution of Relative ULC of the U.S. as compared to a group of eight EU countries (EU-8).[5] The Unit Labor Cost is decomposed into three terms: relative real labor productivity (LP), relative real cost per employee (LC) and relative prices (RP).[6] As explained in the box "Unit Labor Cost (ULC) and Relative ULC Decomposition," values of all variables below (above) 100 mean that countries are better off (worse off) with respect to the U.S.

Figure II.5 highlights that the U.S. outperforms the EU in terms of relative ULC over the entire period considered. There have been only two phases in which European countries have been able to get closer

---

[3] As Rodrik (2006) points out, one of the major determinants of China's rapid growth is the composition of its export basket, which is significantly more sophisticated than what would be normally expected for a country at its income level. Thus China's future growth will be strongly linked to its capacity of trading higher-income products over time. On the other side, India has emphasized skill-intensive rather than labor-intensive manufacturing, and industries with higher-than-average scale (see Kochhar et al, 2006). This, together with an attitudinal shift of the national government towards a pro-business approach, has contributed to build a favorable environment for fast economic growth (see Rodrik and Subramanian, 2004).

[5] Austria, Germany, Denmark, Finland, France, UK, Italy and Sweden.

[6] For a detailed treatment of this decomposition method see sidebar "Unit Labor Cost (ULC) and Relative ULC (RULC) Decomposition".

Table II.5 Nominal labor cost per employee in the pharmaceutical industry (€ thousands at current exchange rate)

Country	Value Added						2003 (U.S. =100)	Annual Growth			
	1980	1985	1990	1995	2001	2003[1]		'80-'85	'85-'90	'90-'95	'95-'03
Austria	14.9	22.3	30.8	45.4	45.9	48.4	54.5	8.1%	6.5%	7.8%	0.8%
Belgium	—	—	—	55.8	61.0	66.7	75.1	—	—	—	2.2%
Germany	17.4	25.2	32.9	48.7	55.7	58.6	66.0	7.4%	5.3%	7.8%	2.3%
Denmark	16.8	23.7	34.7	43.1	58.0	63.2	71.2	6.9%	7.6%	4.3%	4.8%
Spain	—	—	32.5	38.8	48.3	46.6	52.5	—	12.4%	3.5%	2.3%
Finland	10.6	20.6	28.9	29.6	37.3	40.0	45.1	13.3%	6.7%	0.5%	3.8%
France	26.7	33.4	40.0	53.6	70.0	75.8	85.3	4.5%	3.6%	5.8%	4.3%
UK	15.0	27.0	39.0	43.9	89.0	85.6	96.4	11.7%	7.4%	2.4%	8.3%
Greece[2]	—	—	—	16.2	—	—	—	—	—	—	—
Ireland	—	—	22.1	27.6	35.3	39.5	44.5	—	—	4.4%	4.5%
Italy	16.2	25.5	36.4	36.4	49.9	53.4	60.1	9.1%	7.1%	-0.01%	4.8%
Netherlands[3]	—	23.9	24.6	40.6	44.3	48.9	55.1	—	1.1%	10.0%	2.3%
Portugal[4]	—	—	—	22.4	28.9	29.9	33.7	—	—	—	4.1%
Sweden	16.6	26.3	33.0	38.7	54.4	61.7	69.5	9.3%	4.6%	3.2%	5.8%
EU-8[5]	18.1	27.0	36.1	45.4	62.4	65.1	73.3	8.0%	5.8%	4.6%	4.5%
EU-15[6]	—	—	—	44.7	59.8	62.4	70.3	—	—	—	4.2%
U.S.	18.8	52.8	41.5	49.6	93.3	88.8	100.0	20.7%	-4.8%	3.6%	7.3%
Japan	12.6	29.7	35.4	59.1	67.2	59.0	66.5	17.1%	3.5%	10.2%	-0.01%
Czech Rep.[7]	—	—	—	6.1	10.1	10.8	12.2	—	—	—	9.6%
Hungary[8]	—	—	—	10.3	15.4	18.8	21.2	—	—	—	12.1%
Poland[9]	—	—	—	6.7	13.8	—	—	—	—	—	—
Canada	10.4	26.1	23.2	25.9	38.8	—	—	18.4%	-2.4%	2.2%	—
Norway	14.4	24.3	29.1	36.2	50.3	53.9	60.7	10.5%	3.6%	4.4%	5.0%

(1)Projections based on Eurostat survey data (except for Denmark and the U.S.). (2) Period 1995-2000. (3) Period 1987-2003. (4) Period 1996-2003. (5) The EU-8 aggregate includes: Austria, Germany, Denmark, Finland, France, UK, Italy and Sweden. (6) Excluding Greece, Luxembourg and Portugal.(7) Period 2000-2003. (8) Period 1998-2003. (9) Period 1996-2001.

Source: our computations on OECD-STAN, OECD—Main Economic Indicators and GGDC (latest data available)

Figure II.4 Labor cost per employee for the EU in manufacturing and pharmaceuticals *vis-à-vis* the U.S., 1980-2001 (U.S.=100)

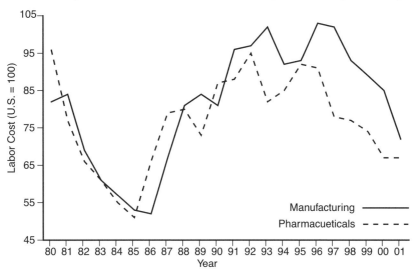

European labor cost has been calculated for the aggregate EU-8, which includes: Austria, Germany, Denmark, Finland, France, UK, Italy and Sweden.

Source: our computations on OECD-STAN, OECD—Main Economic Indicators and GGDC 60-industry database (for pharmaceuticals); GGDC ICOP Database 1997 Benchmark (for manufacturing)

to the U.S.: 1984-1985, and more recently in 2000-2002. U.S. leadership is grounded in its superior labor productivity. On the contrary, the most powerful competitive weapon of Europe has been lower labor cost. While U.S. labor productivity is a sustainable long-term sector-specific advantage that is not easily replicated, EU cost competitiveness is more unstable, subject to general macroeconomic factors and competitive threats by emerging countries.

Indeed, most of the observed volatility in terms of RULC is caused by relative prices, mainly exchange rate fluctuations, but also relative inflation rates. The U-shaped trend of RULC for the period 1980-1987 follows the episode of sharp appreciation and subsequent depreciation of the U.S. dollar against all the main currencies. The smoother episode of U.S. dollar appreciation—begun in 1996 and ended in 2001—caused, together with an increase in labor productivity,[7] the downturn of RULC during that time span, counterbalancing

Unit labor cost (ULC) and Relative ULC (RULC) decomposition

The Unit Labor Cost (ULC) represents the current cost of labor per unit of output and is usually obtained as the ratio of nominal labor cost per employee to real labor productivity. Nominal Labor Cost (hereafter LC) is taken here as total employees compensation over total number of employees, expressed in current prices and converted to a reference currency (USD) using current Exchange Rates (ER).

The Real Labor Productivity (RLP) considers the value added per employee (nominal labor productivity, hereafter LP) and applies the methodology already described in the box "Purchasing Power Parity and International Productivity Comparison", fixing a base year (1997) and expressing all values in PPP with respect to a base currency (USD).

The use of nominal (current price) values for labor compensation and of constant-price values for labor productivity can be better understood when interpreting the unit labor cost measure as an indicator of cost competitiveness. In fact, in this case, we obtain the remuneration per unit of production, expressed in the same unit of measurement independently from the country considered.

This index is particularly useful in calculating the cost competitiveness for tradable goods at the international level, given that labor is a much less mobile factor of production than goods. Indeed, as the price of sticky factors of production is fixed on local markets, it makes sense to consider their cost in nominal terms. On the contrary, for almost perfectly tradable goods we have to express their values upon the prices of a reference country market, since by definition they can be traded on international markets.

Therefore, the ULCs are calculated in the following way:

for European countries:

$$\mathrm{ULC}_{EU}^{\text{€cy}} = \frac{LC}{RLP} = \frac{LC_{EU}^{\text{€cy}}}{LP_{EU}^{\$97}} = \frac{LC_{EU}^{\text{€cy}}/ER^{\text{€cy}/\text{€cy}}}{LP_{EU}^{\text{€cy}} \, DEFL^{\text{€97}/\text{€cy}}/PPP^{\text{€97}/\text{€97}}}$$

for U.S.:

$$\text{ULC}_{US}^{\text{€cy}} = \frac{LC}{RLP} = \frac{LC_{US}^{\text{€cy}}}{LP_{US}^{\$97}} = \frac{LC_{US}^{\text{€cy}}}{LP_{US}^{\$cy}\, \text{DEFL}^{\$97/\$cy}}$$

in formulas:

LC $_{EU}^{\text{€cy}}$ = EU-15 nominal labor cost per employee expressed in current euros;

LC $_{US}^{\$cy}$ = U.S. nominal labor cost per employee expressed in current dollars;

ER $^{\text{€cy}/\$cy}$ = nominal exchange rate dollar/euro;

all other symbols are the same as in box "Purchasing Power Parity and International Productivity Comparison" (page 26).

To compare European countries and the U.S., we compute also the Relative ULC (RULC), which is the percentage ratio of the respective ULC, where the U.S. is the baseline country.

In the following, we show how RULC can be decomposed into three factors: relative real Labor Cost (ratio of LC), relative real labor productivity (ratio of RLP) and Relative Prices (RP).

In formulas (Equation [1]):

$$\text{RULC}_{EU/US}^{\text{cy}} = \frac{\text{ULC}_{EU}^{\text{€cy}}}{\text{ULC}_{US}^{\$cy}} = \frac{LC_{US}^{\text{€cy}}\, \text{DEFL}^{\text{€97}/\text{€cy}}/\text{PPP}^{\text{€97}/\$97}}{LP_{US}^{\$cy}} \bullet$$

$$\frac{LP_{US}^{\text{€cy}}}{LP_{EU}^{\text{€cy}}\, \text{DEFL}^{\text{€97}/\text{€cy}}/\text{PPP}^{\text{€97}/\$97}} \bullet \frac{\text{DEFL}^{\$97/\$cy}\text{PPP}^{\text{€97}/\$97}}{\text{DEFL}^{\text{€97}/\text{€cy}}\, \text{ER}^{\text{€cy}/\$cy}}$$

where symbols have the usual meanings.

This decomposition allows us to fully characterize differences in levels and trends of relative prices in the third term (RP). In Equation [1]:

(a) the first term represents the ratio between real labor costs expressed in USD at constant PPP exchange rates;

(b) the second term is the ratio between real labor productivity expressed in USD at constant PPP exchange rates;

(c) the third term is the overall factor that transforms real values into nominal values.

The RULC decomposition is reported in Table II.5. For the way on which we constructed the decomposition, values of RULC, LC, LP and RP below (above) 100 mean that the country is better off (worse off) with respect to the U.S.

the increase in relative cost per employee. Since 2001 EU RULC relative to the U.S. has started to rise again. This is mainly driven by a worsening of EU labor productivity, even though relative cost per employee has started to decline.

Relative real labor costs were roughly constant until the end of the 1980s. After that, European labor costs went through a period of growth that ended around 1994. Since the second half of the 1990s, labor market reforms introduced by many EU countries started a period of wage moderation, thus stabilizing relative labor costs. Overall, the long-term pattern of the relative labor cost shows an upward time trend.

On the other hand, relative labor productivity exhibited a more erratic behavior, with several upturns and downturns. However, EU performance is consistently worse than that of U.S.

Since 2002, the EU-U.S. competitiveness gap has been widening. The poorer performance of EU pharmaceuticals is mainly the outcome of lower productivity growth, which is not offset by moderation in the growth rate of labor costs.

Table II.6 shows the dynamics of cost competitiveness for the EU-15 countries by reporting a detailed breakdown of their RULC *vis-à-vis* the U.S. for the years 1980, 1990, 1995, 2001, and 2003.

---

[7] Note that, as highlighted in the box, LP above 100 means that a country is worse off with respect to the U.S.

Figure II.5 Temporal evolution of RULC (U.S. = 100) and its components for the EU-8 aggregate[1]

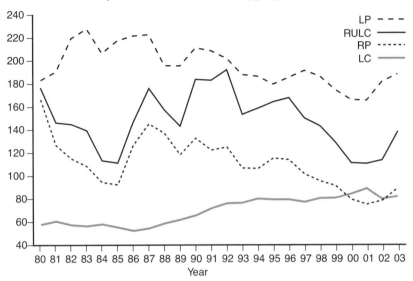

Value of LP higher than 100 means a lower labor productivity in Europe than in the U.S., as well as lower values of RULC, LC and RP indicate, respectively, lower values of relative unit labor cost, real labor cost and relative prices than in the U.S.

(1) The EU-8 aggregate includes: Austria, Germany, Denmark, Finland, France, UK, Italy and Sweden (80 percent of EU-15 value added in pharmaceuticals in 2000). Values for 2002 and 2003 have been obtained as projections from Eurostat survey data (except for Denmark and the U.S.).

Source: our computations on OECD-STAN, OECD—Main Economic Indicators, Eurostat and GGDC (latest data available)

Despite higher labor costs, the U.S. maintains its cost competitiveness, thanks to productivity gains.

Among EU countries, the best performers in 2003 in terms of RULC were scored by Ireland (42.1), Sweden (65.3), and Belgium (98.7), with ULC levels close to those of the U.S., significantly improving their RULC over the period considered. Not by chance, Ireland, Belgium and Sweden are among the main recipients of foreign direct investments, mostly from the U.S. Notably, these countries succeeded in keeping labor costs under control while experiencing rates of productivity growth higher than the average (see Table II.5). Therefore, their good performances are less dependent on exchange rate movements and, in a sense, motivate foreign investments, compared to their EU partners. In recent years other countries showed RULC levels close to or below the U.S., namely France

(112.2 in 2003; 94.1 in 2001), Denmark (116.3 in 2003; 79.8 in 2001), and the Netherlands (74.8 in 2003; 116.7 in 2001).

Germany and Italy still show productivity levels which are less than half that of the U.S., although Italy has been more successful than the EU average in adopting wage moderation policies. As for the UK, its modest RULC performance is due more to its failure to contain labor costs (higher than in the U.S. in real terms) than to negative productivity performances. On the contrary, UK productivity has been growing faster than the EU average.

In conclusion, the European scenario is quite heterogeneous. On the one side there is a group of countries, notably northern European EU member states (and to a lesser extent France and UK), that greatly increased their productivity. On the other side, Germany, Italy, Spain and Greece have strived to compete mainly through exchange rate depreciation and labor cost containment, but have been performing poorly in terms of productivity levels and growth rates. As dramatically testified by the experience of transition economies, this pattern is not sustainable in the long run, since countries with low labor costs and rapidly increasing productivity levels could emerge, and the less favorable exchange rate no longer compensates for lower labor productivity levels. Indeed, since 2002, under the effect of the appreciation of the euro and the U.S. productivity revival, Europe has lost further ground relative to the U.S.

II.4   Growth Decomposition and Total Factor Productivity

Table II.7 shows the level of capitalization[8] for the EU-15 countries relative to the U.S. in 1980-2003. Due to lack of data, we are not able to make comparisons along the entire period for all EU-15 countries, but only for a subset of them (Germany, France and UK, included in the aggregate EU-3). Since the 1990s, we also report an aggregate consisting of 10 countries (EU-10):[9] Austria, Belgium, Germany, Finland, France, UK, Ireland, Italy, Netherlands, and Sweden.

---

[8] Capital per employee expressed in standard efficiency units (built following the method described in the box "Growth decomposition and TFP") and converted to PPP USD by using PPP rates for Gross Fixed Capital Formation (source: OECD).

[9] Note that in general EU-10 denotes the group of the new member states; only in this section we use this label referring to Austria, Belgium, Germany, Finland, France, UK, Ireland, Italy, Netherlands, and Sweden.

Table II.6 Relative unit labor cost in the pharmaceutical industry (U.S.=100) and its decomposition[1,2]

	1980				1990				1995				2001				2003[2]			
	RULC	LP	LC	RP	RULC	LP	LC	RP	RULC	LP	LC	RP	RULC	LP	LC	RP	RULC	LP	LC	RP
Austria	185.2	234.2	46.5	170.2	185.1	249.0	51.8	143.6	185.5	202.5	69.2	132.4	142.7	289.8	61.7	79.7	132.1	242.3	54.8	99.5
Belgium	—	—	—	—	—	—	—	—	151.9	135.1	91.4	123.1	74.9	114.5	95.0	68.9	98.7	131.4	88.7	84.7
Germany	167.7	180.9	63.9	145.2	230.0	289.6	54.7	145.2	224.3	228.4	74.1	132.5	142.4	238.7	77.6	76.9	183.9	278.5	69.7	94.7
Denmark	129.7	144.9	80.2	111.7	216.2	258.3	56.7	147.5	165.5	190.3	65.9	131.9	79.8	128.4	86.5	71.9	116.3	163.2	68.2	104.5
Spain	—	—	—	—	161.8	206.4	66.8	117.4	150.0	191.6	87.9	89.1	119.4	230.9	80.9	63.9	151.2	288.0	63.5	82.6
Finland	74.1	131.4	40.3	140.0	163.1	234.4	43.3	160.8	157.4	264.0	46.3	128.8	110.9	277.6	51.1	78.2	141.9	314.5	49.4	91.2
France	324.4	228.8	51.8	273.5	179.0	185.7	75.2	128.2	153.4	141.9	91.9	117.6	94.1	125.5	109.0	68.8	112.2	131.5	106.3	80.3
UK	141.1	176.4	54.7	146.2	188.2	200.4	70.1	133.9	153.8	173.7	81.8	108.2	125.8	131.9	116.5	81.8	163.1	169.2	107.3	89.8
Greece[3]	—	—	—	—	—	—	—	—	228.3	700.5	25.6	127.4	177.8	829.6	25.2	85.0	—	—	—	—
Ireland	—	—	—	—	106.5	199.6	36.4	146.8	65.1	117.0	43.2	128.6	45.3	119.7	38.7	97.6	42.1	94.7	41.3	107.8
Italy	146.1	169.9	55.7	154.5	148.6	169.4	73.9	118.6	135.0	184.0	80.4	91.3	102.4	191.5	73.4	72.9	137.2	228.3	66.8	90.0
Netherlands	—	—	—	—	158.1	266.3	57.0	104.1	129.7	158.5	72.5	112.8	74.8	157.6	82.5	57.5	116.7	211.6	88.9	62.0
Sweden	153.7	174.6	61.8	142.4	156.4	196.6	56.5	140.8	91.1	116.6	68.6	114.0	62.4	107.1	82.5	70.6	65.3	93.9	82.8	83.9
EU-8[4]	176.3	183.2	57.8	164.7	183.8	211.3	65.6	132.0	164.5	179.6	79.3	114.9	110.6	165.6	89.0	74.6	138.1	188.4	82.1	88.7
EU-15[5]	—	—	—	—	—	—	—	—	159.2	176.4	79.8	113.4	105.7	165.1	87.1	73.7	131.5	187.1	80.0	88.2
U.S.	100.0	100.0	100.0	100.0	100.0	100.0	100.0	100.0	100.0	100.0	100.0	100.0	100.0	100.0	100.0	100.0	100.0	100.0	100.0	100.0

A value of LP higher than 100 means a lower labor productivity than in the U.S. Lower values of RULC, LC and RP indicate, respectively, lower values of relative unit labor cost, real labor cost and relative prices than in the U.S. (1) See box "Unit labor cost (ULC) and relative ULC decomposition". Changes of relative prices represent the part of variations of value added that does not depend on changes in production volumes. (2) Projections based on Eurostat survey data (Except for Denmark and the U.S. (3) Data available in 2000. (4) The EU-8 aggregate includes: Austria, Germany, Denmark, Finland, France, UK, Italy and Sweden. (5) Excluding Greece, Luxembourg and Portugal.

Source: our computations on OECD-STAN, OECD—Main Economic Indicators, Eurostat and GGDC (last data available).

Reading key: RULC = relative unit labor cost × 100 (equal to the product of LP×LC×RP, see box "Unit labor cost (ULC) and relative ULC decomposition").
LP = relative real labor productivity at constant PPP dollars (U.S. at the numerator) × 100. **LC** = relative real labor cost at constant PPP dollars (U.S. at the denominator) × 100.
RP = overall relative price factor × 100

With few exceptions (e.g. France and Belgium), capital accumulation occurred in the U.S. at consistently higher rates than in the EU. In 2003, capital per employee in the U.S. was 56.7 percent above the EU-10 aggregate level. Moreover, the growth rate of capital per employee was 2.1 percentage points higher (in the period 1995-2003). From 1990 to 2003 the U.S. capital stock almost doubled in real terms.

Interesting differences emerge by splitting the EU-10 aggregate into two groups of countries based on their productivity performances: EU-H and EU-L. EU-H "Tigers" includes those countries with high productivity growth (Belgium, France, UK, Ireland and Sweden), while EU-L "Tortoises" is the group of low productivity growth countries (Austria, Germany, Finland, Italy and Netherlands). The first set of countries enjoyed an average growth rate of capital per employee comparable to that of the U.S. in the first half of the 1990s. Thereafter (over the period 1995-2003), they lost some ground. This was caused by the slowdown in capital accumulation in 2002-2003. However, the EU-H growth rate still remained fairly above the EU-10 and the EU-L levels.

Within the EU-H group, the Belgian capital growth rate was five percentage points higher than that of the U.S. in the period 1995-2003, thanks to foreign direct investments, especially from the U.S. (see Chapter III).[10] Sweden was the only country with comparable levels of capital per employee with respect to the U.S. in 2003. On the contrary, having been the target of huge capital investments in the past, Ireland presented negative accumulation rates, substituting labor for capital.

Table II.8 reports the factors remuneration share on production value. These data substantially confirm the picture thus far. The U.S. had the highest non-labor inputs shares[11] (30.9 percent of production in 1996-2003) together with the northern EU countries (Ireland, Sweden, Belgium and Denmark). On the contrary, the EU-L aggregate showed a lower share of non-labor inputs equal to 14.5 percent of production in

---

[10] In 2005, the ratio of FDI inward (outward) stocks to the Belgian's GDP reached 132.3 (103.8) percent as compared to 33.5 (40.7) percent for the EU (UNCTAD, 2006).

[11] Given the well-known problems in the correct measurement of capital intensity, this variable can be used as another proxy for the relative intensity of production inputs. However, one should be aware that also this variable has its limits: cross-country differences in relative input prices can seriously bias international comparisons.

Table II.7   Capital per employee in the pharmaceutical industry (1997-PPP € thousands)

Country	Capital per Employee 1980	1985	1990	1995	2001	2003[1]	2003 (U.S. =100)	Annual Growth '80-'85	'85-'90	'90-'95	'95-'03
Austria	44.6	40.7	59.5	66.6	82.5	90.3	78.2	-1.8%	7.9%	3.6%	*3.9%*
Belgium	—	—	—	30.5	60.6	62.2	53.9	—	—	11.5%	*9.3%*
Germany	24.8	29.5	33.9	45.7	55.7	56.7	49.1	3.5%	2.8%	3.3%	*2.7%*
Finland	71.2	69.7	60.7	55.4	52.6	66.4	57.5	-0.4%	-2.7%	-0.9%	*2.3%*
France	15.9	21.1	32.3	48.6	62	69.6	60.2	5.8%	8.9%	4.1%	*4.6%*
UK	46.2	55.6	66.3	79.9	93.9	91.7	79.4	3.8%	3.6%	2.7%	*1.7%*
Ireland	—	—	—	127.1	90.1	96.5	83.5	—	—	-5.7%	*-3.4%*
Italy	—	—	—	80.2	79.3	81.1	70.2	—	—	-0.2%	*0.1%*
Netherlands[2]	—	—	47.2	57.8	57.2	69.1	59.8	—	—	-0.2%	*2.3%*
Sweden	—	—	—	89.6	108.3	106.6	92.2	—	—	3.2%	*2.2%*
EU-3[3]	29	34.8	42.4	55.9	67.1	68.9	59.6	3.7%	4.0%	3.0%	*2.6%*
EU-10[4]	—	—	—	62.2	71.4	73.8	63.8	—	—	2.3%	*2.2%*
EU-H[5]	—	—	—	65.6	79.4	82	71	—	—	3.2%	*2.8%*
EU-L[6]	—	—	—	59.4	65	67.3	58.2	—	—	1.5%	*1.6%*
U.S.	35.5	47.8	59.7	82.3	99.6	115.5	100	6.1%	4.5%	3.2%	*4.3%*
Canada	20.1	28.2	36.6	54.9	52.3	57.9	50.2	7.0%	5.4%	-0.8%	*0.7%*
Norway	21.4	26.4	45.4	42.8	50.6	55.5	48	4.3%	11.5%	2.8%	*3.3%*

(1) Projections based on Eurostat survey data (except for Denmark and the U.S.) (2) 1987-1990 instead of 1986-1990. (3) The EU-3 aggregate includes Germany, France and UK (4) The EU-10 aggregate includes: Austria, Belgium, Germany, Finland, France, UK, Ireland, Italy, Netherlands and Sweden. (5) The EU-H aggregate includes: Belgium, France, UK, Ireland and Sweden. (6) The EU-L aggregate includes: Austria, Germany, Finland, Italy and Netherlands.

Source: our calculations on OECD-STAN, OECD—Main Economic Indicators, Eurostat and GGDC (latest data available)

the period 1996-2003. These marked differences between the U.S. and the EU-H on one side, and the EU-L on the other, mostly translate into differences in the share of production value added, while the share of labor-inputs displays much lower variation. The results confirm the evidence presented in GOP (2000), pointing out the presence in the EU-L aggregate of a large number of fringe companies specialized in low value added activities, mainly in manufacturing and commercialization of products licensed in by foreign companies.

Analogously, the EU-H countries displayed a share of labor inputs close to the U.S. share (19.3 and 19 percent respectively in 2003),

Table II.8   Share of labor and non-labor inputs on production value (1981-2003)

	1981-1985			1986-1990			1991-1995			1996-2003[1]		
	LI	NLI	VA	LI	NLI	VA	LI	NLI	VA	LI	NLI	VA
Austria	24.9	8.1	33.0	23.5	15.6	39.1	24.4	18.6	42.9	20.7	17.3	38.0
Belgium	—	—	—	—	—	—	—	—	—	18.6	23.6	42.2
Germany	33.5	12.1	45.6	31.4	14.4	45.8	31.8	13.2	44.9	28.6	12.1	40.7
Denmark	28.6	13.6	42.2	31.4	17.7	49.1	27.4	24.5	52.0	21.0	27.9	48.9
Spain	—	—	—	25.5	15.4	41.0	25.8	13.5	39.4	22.6	11.1	33.7
Finland	21.9	41.6	63.4	24.9	31.8	56.7	25.4	30.1	55.6	23.4	22.8	46.2
France	21.4	8.9	30.3	18.6	13.0	31.5	17.7	12.5	30.2	16.9	16.2	33.1
UK	29.8	17.8	47.7	31.8	20.3	52.1	28.4	19.0	47.4	26.4	18.8	45.2
Greece[2]	—	—	—	—	—	—	—	—	—	—	—	—
Ireland	—	—	—	—	—	—	13.6	36.7	50.4	8.6	44.6	53.2
Italy	18.5	13.9	32.4	19.0	18.1	37.0	21.8	15.3	37.2	21.5	18.0	39.5
Netherlands[3]	—	—	—	18.7	11.7	30.4	17.1	14.9	32.0	11.3	11.3	22.6
Sweden	32.8	18.1	50.9	27.9	28.4	56.3	18.6	35.1	53.7	17.3	34.8	52.1
EU-8[4]	25.3	13.0	38.3	24.4	16.5	40.9	24.1	15.9	40.0	22.5	17.6	40.1
EU-15[5]	—	—	—	—	—	—	23.9	16.1	40.0	21.3	18.0	39.3
EU-10[6]	—	—	—	—	—	—	23.7	16.1	39.8	21.2	18.2	39.4
EU-H[7]	—	—	—	—	—	—	21.5	17.4	39.0	19.3	21.2	40.5
EU-L[8]	—	—	—	—	—	—	26.1	14.7	40.7	23.5	14.5	38.0
U.S.	23.6	20.3	43.9	20.9	22.1	43.0	19.2	28.0	47.2	19.0	30.9	49.8

Value of non labor inputs computed as total value added (VA) minus personnel costs (LI).

(1) Projections based on Eurostat survey data (except for Denmark and the U.S). (2)1996-2000 instead of 1996-2001. (3) 1987-1990 instead of 1986-1990. (4) The EU-8 aggregate includes: Austria, Germany, Denmark, Finland, France, UK, Italy and Sweden. (5) Excluding Greece, Luxembourg and Portugal (6) The EU-10 aggregate includes: Austria, Belgium, Germany, Finland, France, UK, Ireland, Italy, Netherlands and Sweden. (7) The EU-H aggregate includes: Belgium, France, UK, Ireland and Sweden. (8) The EU-L aggregate includes: Austria, Germany, Finland, Italy and Netherlands.

Source: our calculations on OECD-STAN, OECD—Main Economic Indicators, Eurostat and GGDC (latest data available)

while the EU-L countries showed higher labor intensity (23.5 percent in 2003).

Overall, the U.S. and the small northern EU members seem to be heading for a highly capital intensive production model.

Across European countries, France shows an even distribution between labor and non-labor inputs, while Italy and the UK have a sizable capital stock but their current capital accumulation rates are too low. Finally, Germany is characterized by low capital share.

The relevant differences between the EU and the U.S. call for a deeper analysis of the factors that may drive productivity and growth in the drug industry. To do that, we rely on traditional growth accounting techniques to estimate the contribution of each factor to valued-added growth and to the growth of labor productivity (see box "Growth decomposition and the TFP"). Generally speaking, this methodology aims at decomposing economic growth by considering the production side of the economy, so to decompose the growth of aggregate output into contributions from growth in factor inputs (capital, labor and other factors) and from improvements in technology and the organization of production factors.

Growth decomposition sheds some light on the differences within Europe, suggesting some of the reasons behind the fast growth recently experienced by the northern European countries, notably Ireland, Sweden and Belgium, in comparison with the poor performance of the others, Germany in particular.

Results are summarized in Tables II.9-10. Table II.9 reports the growth rates of the production and of its components (labor, capital and the Solow residual) from 1982 to 2003. Table II.10 focuses on the period 1996-2003, describing the contribution of each input to the output growth.[12]

Table II.9 shows that for the period 1996 to 2003 the average annual output growth rate in the EU-10[13] amounted to 7.2 percent, slightly

---

[12] When calculating TFP for sub-sectors of the economy usually the methodology followed is the "value-added growth decomposition", where value-added substitutes for output. See box "*Growth decomposition and TFP*," for more details.

[13] The EU-10 aggregate includes the following countries: Austria, Belgium, Germany, Finland, France, UK, Ireland, Italy, Netherlands and Sweden.

lower than the U.S. rate (8 percent). In addition, the labor growth rates are really close (1.2 percent in EU-10 vs. 1.6 percent in the U.S.), while both capital growth and total factor productivity (TFP) tend to diverge. In particular, from 1996 to 2003, the EU-10 experienced a higher increase in TFP than the U.S. (5 vs. 3.8 percent), while the opposite occurred for capital growth (3.4 vs. 5.8 percent).

Table II.10 shows that TFP improvements are essential for production growth, both in the EU and in the U.S. However, the two geographical areas present a different pattern: whereas in the U.S. the contributions to production growth given by TFP and capital are similar (respectively 3.8 percent-column d—and 3.6 percent-column c), for Europe TFP is by far the most important factor. In both regions, labor contribution is minor, less than 1 percent (column b).

A complementary view on the main determinants of the output growth is provided by the decomposition the labor productivity growth (column e) into growth of capital per worker (or capital deepening, column f) and total factor productivity (column g). According to the results in Table II.10, both in the U.S. and in the EU-10 labor productivity growth has been mostly the outcome of a significant growth of total factor productivity (TFP). This is especially true for EU-10. The U.S. experienced a significant process of capital accumulation too (2.6 percent vs. 1.0 percent in Europe).

While for the U.S. both investments in physical capital and general technological progress matter, in Europe the major driver of output growth is TFP.

The European aggregate conceals the presence of strong cross-country variations. Focusing on the previously defined aggregates, EU-H and EU-L, we note that:

1. In 1996-2003 the EU-H aggregate experienced significant productivity gains (7.7 percent), associated with both high capital accumulation (1.4) and very high TFP growth (6.3 percent). In particular, it is likely that the high value of TFP growth is the result of the past capital investments activity. Within the EU-H aggregate, Belgium, Sweden and Ireland present the highest capital contribution to the overall output growth (6.8, 3.8 and 2.6 percent respectively). However, according also to figures in Table II.7, Ireland shows a nega-

Table II.9   Production, labor, capital and TFP growth, 1982-2003 percent (%)[1,2]

	1982-1990				1991-1995				1996-2003[2]			
	Pro	Lab	Cap	TFP	Pro	Lab	Cap	TFP	Pro	Lab	Cap	TFP
	$\dot{Y}$	$\dot{L}$	$\dot{K}$	$\dot{A}$	$\dot{Y}$	$\dot{L}$	$\dot{K}$	$\dot{A}$	$\dot{Y}$	$\dot{L}$	$\dot{K}$	$\dot{A}$
Austria	10.2	3.5	6.5	5.3	7.4	1.1	3.4	5.2	4.7	0.5	4.3	2.6
Belgium	—	—	—	—	—	—	—	—	10.4	3.6	12.6	2.1
Germany	3.6	1.0	4.5	1.5	5.5	-1.3	4.7	5.2	5.7	1.8	4.5	3.2
Finland	3.0	3.5	1.8	0.5	0.2	0.5	-1.3	0.7	3.6	-0.7	1.6	3.3
France	10.6	1.8	9.7	5.9	7.3	-0.2	8.0	4.2	7.5	0.1	4.6	5.2
UK	6.7	0.1	4.1	5.1	3.9	-1.1	2.7	3.6	6.3	-0.4	1.3	6.1
Ireland	—	—	—	—	—	—	—	—	15.5	6.4	3.0	11.8
Italy	—	—	—	—	—	—	—	—	5.2	1.4	1.6	3.7
Netherlands	—	—	—	—	11.9	-0.6	3.4	10.7	4.1	1.2	3.5	2.1
Sweden	—	—	—	—	—	—	—	—	12.9	3.7	5.9	7.8
EU-3[3]	6.48	1.0	5.2	4.1	5.6	-1.0	4.6	4.7	6.6	0.7	3.4	4.8
EU-10[4]	—	—	—	—	—	—	—	—	7.2	1.2	3.4	5.0
EU-H[5]	—	—	—	—	—	—	—	—	8.6	0.9	3.7	6.3
EU-L[6]	—	—	—	—	—	—	—	—	5.3	1.5	3.1	3.2
U.S.	7.6	0.9	6.6	4.0	5.0	2.9	9.4	-1.7	8.0	1.6	5.8	3.8

(1) See the box "Growth Decomposition and TFP" for a description of the methodology applied to decompose the growth of output. (2)Projections based on Eurostat survey data (except for Denmark and the U.S.). (3) The EU-3 aggregate includes Germany, France and UK (4) The EU-10 aggregate includes: Austria, Belgium, Germany, Finland, France, UK, Ireland, Italy, Netherlands and Sweden. (5) The EU-H aggregate includes: Belgium, France, UK, Ireland and Sweden. (6) The EU-L aggregate includes: Austria, Germany, Finland, Italy and Netherlands.

Source: our computations on OECD-STAN, OECD—Main Economic Indicators and GGDC (latest data available)

Reading key: **Pro** = Production, **Lab** = Labor, **Cap** = Capital, **TFP** = Total Factor Productivity

tive capital accumulation, i.e. a negative growth of capital per worker. This is probably due to the slow substitution of labor for capital.

2. In contrast with the previous group of countries, the EU-L aggregate has experienced lower growth of output per worker (3.8 percent), mostly because of the negative performance of Germany and Italy. As well as for EU-H countries, more than

Table II.10   Factors contribution to output growth and to labor productivity growth (1996-2003)[1,2]

	(a)	(b)		(c)		(d)	(e) value added per worker	(f) capital deep-ing	(g)
	ouput growth	labor contri-bution	labor share	capital contri-bution	capital share	TFP			TFP
	$\dot{Y}$	$(1-\alpha)\dot{L}$	$(1-\alpha)$	$\alpha\dot{K}$	α	$\dot{A}$	$\dot{Y}-\dot{L}$	$\alpha(\dot{K}-\dot{L})$	$\dot{A}$
Austria	4.7	0.2	0.6	1.9	0.5	2.6	4.2	1.6	2.6
Belgium	10.4	1.5	0.4	6.8	0.6	2.1	6.8	4.7	2.1
Germany	5.7	1.2	0.7	1.3	0.3	3.2	4.0	0.8	3.2
Finland	3.6	-0.4	0.5	0.7	0.5	3.3	4.3	1.0	3.3
France	7.5	0.1	0.5	2.3	0.5	5.2	7.4	2.2	5.2
UK	6.3	-0.3	0.6	0.6	0.4	6.1	6.8	0.7	6.1
Ireland	15.5	1.2	0.2	2.6	0.8	11.8	9.1	-2.7	11.8
Italy	5.2	0.8	0.6	0.7	0.5	3.7	3.7	0.1	3.7
Netherlands	4.1	0.5	0.5	1.5	0.5	2.1	2.8	0.8	2.1
Sweden	12.9	1.3	0.3	3.8	0.6	7.8	9.1	1.4	7.8
EU-3[3]	6.6	0.4	0.6	1.3	0.4	4.8	5.8	1.0	4.8
EU-10[4]	7.2	0.7	0.5	1.5	0.5	5.0	5.9	1.0	5.0
EU-H[5]	8.6	0.4	0.5	1.9	0.5	6.3	7.7	1.4	6.3
EU-L[6]	5.3	0.9	0.6	1.2	0.4	3.2	3.8	0.6	3.2
U.S.	8.0	0.6	0.4	3.6	0.6	3.8	6.4	2.6	3.8

$(a) = (b) + (c) + (d)$ $\qquad$ $(e) = (f) + (g)$

(1) See the box "Growth Decomposition and TFP" for a description of the methodology applied for decomposing output growth. (2) Projections based on Eurostat survey data (except for Denmark and the U.S). (3) The EU-3 aggregate includes Germany, France and UK (4) The EU-10 aggregate includes: Austria, Belgium, Germany, Finland, France, UK, Ireland, Italy, Netherlands and Sweden. (5) The EU-H aggregate includes: Belgium, France, UK, Ireland and Sweden. (6) The EU-L aggregate includes: Austria, Germany, Finland, Italy and Netherlands.

Source: our computations on OECD-STAN, OECD—Main Economic Indicators, Eurostat and GGDC (latest data available)

80 percent of labor productivity growth is explained by TFP growth. However, given the low values for capital accumulation it is reasonable to expect for the foreseeable future a further deterioration of labor productivity and TFP growth.

Figure II.6 shows the decomposition of the value added growth for the three leading EU countries in pharmaceuticals (France, Germany and UK), plus the U.S. The results have been obtained by applying a Hodrick-Prescott filter to the original series in order to eliminate short-term fluctuations.

Some differences emerge among leading EU countries.

Over the 1980s, France experienced a decreasing trend in both labor productivity and TFP growth while capital accumulation increased. The successive downturn in capital accumulation in the following decade was counterbalanced by an upswing in TFP growth (probably due to the effect of past investment efforts) therefore contributing to the stabilization of the labor productivity trend.

Both Germany and the UK experienced an increase in valued added during the 1980s, whereas the opposite occurs during the 1990s. Since 2000, however, their patterns seem to diverge. In Germany, employment growth reflects the non-decreasing trend in value added growth, while TFP growth follows a roughly stable path and capital accumulation declines. On the contrary, in the UK the evolution of labor productivity as well as TFP growth have caused a downward sloping trend of value added growth. Capital accumulation is aslo declining.

As far as employment growth is concerned, France, Germany, and the UK display similar trends. In fact, all of them are characterized by declining (even negative) growth employment rates between the end of the 1980s and the first half of the 1990s. This period has been affected by rising labor costs, which ended also thanks to the reforms of the labor market introduced later on. In the following period, indeed, employment growth restarts due to wage moderation policies. Moreover, the dynamics of employment growth follows the profile of the economic cycle, as measured by value added growth rate. Indeed, value added growth displays a slowdown in the first half of the 1990s in all the countries considered, in coincidence with the economic crisis experienced by the U.S. in the same period (see Blanchard, 1993). In the following period, employment growth rate increases.

The U.S. decomposition sums up the evidence emerging in the previous sections, namely higher rates of TFP growth and labor productivity since the second half of the 1990s. During the same period, a slowdown

Growth decomposition and TFP

Total Factor Productivity (TFP) growth explains the part of production growth unaccounted by the growth of labor and capital (Solow, 1957). TFP is thus a "measure of our ignorance," with ample scope for measurement error. It may represent the contribution of various kinds of externalities, such as those that may generate from technological, institutional and organizational change.

As data quality increases, allowing to include labor quality (i.e. human capital) and different types of capital (like ICT capital) to our input measures, then TFP growth comes to represent ideally the contribution of disembodied knowledge to production's growth.

TFP growth is obtained by employing the usual growth accounting procedure (see for instance Jorgenson and Griliches, 1967). Suppose that real output could be represented by the mean of a Cobb-Douglas production function

$$Y_t = A_t K_t^\alpha L_t^{1-\alpha} \quad \text{[eq. 1]},$$

where K_t is the capital stock at time t, L_t is the amount of workers at time t and A_t a factor of scale capturing various kinds of externalities at time t, and primarily technological progress; by taking the logarithm and the time differences, the above equation becomes:

$$y_t - y_{t-1} = a_t - a_{t-1} = \alpha(k_t - k_{t-1}) + (1-\alpha)(l_t - l_{t-1}) \quad \text{[eq. 2]},$$

where lowercase letters represent the natural logarithm of the variables in equation [1].

In a standard optimization problem where factors of production are chosen in a way to minimize cost subject to the production function [1], the factors of production are compensated in an amount equal to their productivity.

Therefore, keeping in mind that $\ln X_t - \ln X_{t-1} \cong \dot{X}_t$ equation [2] could be rewritten as:

$\dot{Y}_t = \dot{A}_t + \alpha \dot{K}_t + (1-\alpha)\dot{L}_t$ [eq. *3*],

where $\alpha = \dfrac{\mu K}{pY}$ and $(1-\alpha) = \dfrac{wL}{pY}$, with μ, w respectively the unit return for capital and work, and p the output price.

The term $\dot{A}$, namely the rate of growth of TFP, is calculated as a residual by subtracting from the output growth $(\dot{Y}_t)$ the other two terms in equation [3].

Another useful decomposition is given by rearranging equation [3] in the following way:

$\dot{Y}_t - \dot{L} = \alpha(\dot{K}_t - \dot{L}_t) + \dot{A}_t$ [eq. *4*]

where the term on the left hand side represents labor productivity growth and the terms on the right hand side its decomposition in capital deepening and TFP growth.

When calculating TFP for sub-sectors of the economy, also intermediate inputs should be considered as factors of production in equation [1]-[4]. When measures for these intermediate inputs are not available, a "value-added growth decomposition" can be nevertheless obtained, where the value added takes the place of production as Y_t in equation [1].

In order to obtain the series of TFP growth, we estimate equation [3].

First, we use the series of the share of employees compensation to value added as a proxy for $(1-\alpha)$ over time. Next, we take the growth rate in the number of employees as a measure of labor growth rate. Finally, in order to obtain the time series for capital, we use the perpetual inventory method from the investment series after deflating by the appropriate index (from OECD-STAN)[1].

---

[1] The perpetual inventory method assumes a time formation path for capital like $K_t = I_t + (1-\delta)K_{t-1}$, with a depreciation rate of capital (δ) of 8 percent per annum; the stock of capital of the initial year is reconstructed as $K_0 = I_0/(\gamma + \delta)$, using, as a pre-sample net growth rate of capital (γ), a growth rate of 5 percent. The values for δ and γ are derived from commonly accepted empirical results on the machineries deterioration and the average net rate of investment. See for instance Crepon et al (1998).

in capital accumulation also emerged. This negative trend reversed only from the end of the 1990s. Employment growth rate remains almost stable since the end of the 1980s apart from a small decrease and a subsequent quick recovering in the second half of the 1990s.

This empirical evidence for the U.S. is in line with our main findings on R&D productivity. In fact, low R&D productivity might be the main cause of meager U.S. TFP performances (see Chapter IV).

Investments in R&D and in General Purpose Technologies represent a relevant component of U.S. fixed capital formation in pharmaceuticals (see GCP, 2000).[14] This explains why, in the U.S., TFP, together with real capital accumulation, is the most important driver in output growth (see Table II.8 and II.9).

Moreover, firms need some time to implement organizational changes to exploit at best general-purpose innovation (R&D output). This "transition" phase started at the beginning of the 1990s. It is characterized by a larger amount of capital and labor inputs, while the expected increase in output will occur only later on. Therefore, TFP growth turns out to be lower during the transition phase. In other words, the effect of R&D investments on output growth, captured by TFP, shows up with delay (see David, 1990 and Yang-Brynjolfsson, 2001). Hence, current R&D efforts will be translated into R&D output and in turn in productivity growth in the future. As described in Chapter IV, the slowdown that affects market growth rates for innovative products from the mid-1990s, suggests that the U.S. business model is probably still in transition and the fruits of General Purpose (Post) Genomics Technologies are yet to come.

II.5   The Role of Institutions

As previously discussed, TFP can be thought of as a measure of general progress. The non-measurable factors in TFP include innovations, as well as the application of improvements in general knowledge and in the organization of production. As the empirical literature shows (McKinsey 2001, van Ark *et al.* 2002), different diffusion rates and different impact on productivity of investment in Information and

---

[14] See also Table IV.2: the R&D ratio in the U.S. during the period 1991-1995 was 2.50, 1.28 percent higher than in 1986-1990.

Figure II.6   Decomposition of value added trend growth for the U.S., France, Germany and UK

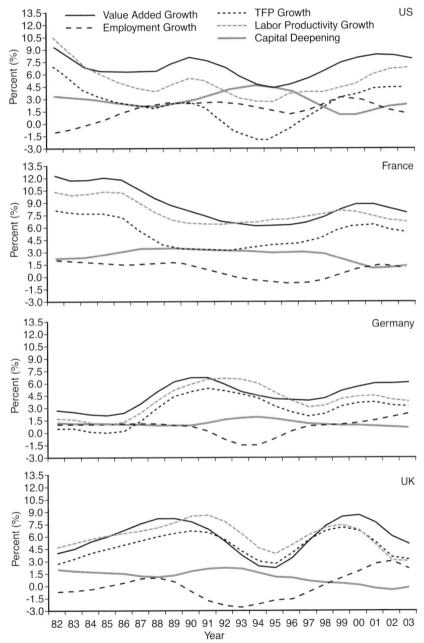

Source: our computations on Eurostat (NewCronos) and U.S. Census Bureau (latest data available).

Communication Technologies are among the main causes of the recent U.S.-EU productivity gap.

In particular, it was found that the difference in overall economy wide productivity stems from the high productivity gains achieved by the U.S. economy in three intensive ICT user services, namely: wholesale trade, retail trade, and financial services. Together, they accounted for two thirds of U.S. productivity growth in the second half of the 1990s. This performance has been achieved thanks to the introduction of ICT technologies accompanied by effective organizational changes and by the exploitation of economies of scale.

Since TFP growth is measured as a residual, it contains an array of effects such as cyclical components, pure changes in efficiency, and measurement errors. TFP also captures country heterogeneity in terms of institutions, through their influence on regulatory policies and hence on competition (Alesina *et al.*, 2005). The findings of Alesina *et al.* (2005) suggest that efficient regulatory reforms lead to increased investment of firms, so that effects of competition can work through increased capital accumulation as well as through TFP growth. Hence, strong competition and deregulation in the U.S. could also explain why the United States shows a more balanced model of productivity growth than the EU, since both technological progress and capital accumulation matter.

In this context, the intervention of some European governments into the market for pharmaceuticals, in particular through price controls and restrictions on patent protection, can prevent the higher growth rates of capital accumulation that would lead the EU towards a more sustainable model of production growth.

Issues about competition and regulation will be further analyzed in Chapter V, while in the following we discuss the role played by other institutional aspects in explaining the EU-U.S. gap.

Financing and tax incentives for firms, the availability of venture capital to start new R&D projects and tax incentives to encourage capital formation and stimulate R&D in the private sector are very important. The U.S. stock market and financial institutions certainly have a relevant role.[15] Indeed, advanced rules for financial disclosure

---

[15] For a detailed analysis of the institutional factors behind the EU-U.S. productivity gap see Gordon (2004).

and access to internal information by equity analysts led ultimately to the creation of a solid network of innovation seeking finance specialists, resulting in turn in a flourishing venture capital industry. Even after the stock market crash such expertise is still based mainly in the U.S., seeking out the next round of innovation.

Another important factor in re-establishing U.S. industrial leadership is its competitive university system, and the close interplay among universities, public research centers, and companies, mainly in hi-tech sectors. The interplay among different institutions has been often supported by public intervention through a variety of governmental agencies (i.e. NSF, NIH, DoD), acting as catalysts of innovation, in particular through "mission oriented" research programs financed through competitive research and procurement schemes (see Stokes, 1996). Differently from public intervention in Europe, which awards the largest share of financing to the whole structure (being a university or a company), in the U.S. funding is more strictly linked to performance and assigned to individual researchers through a peer-reviewed process.

Adequately trained scientific and technical personnel (skilled labor force) are vital to any country's industrial competitiveness. To a certain extent, all countries with a good university system in a field have also a good supply of well-trained people in that field, however, that is not sufficient to guarantee country competitiveness. The EU institutional framework should be able also to promote vertical labor mobility and career patterns for high skilled human capital. Otherwise, the internationalization of labor markets would imply the migration of talents to the U.S. (brain-drain effect).

Finally, the low level of regulation (and of unionization) in the U.S. labor market helps also to guarantee horizontal labor mobility from sectors in crisis to high growth sectors in a more effective way than in Europe.

Other important institutional differences with Europe can be identified in a long tradition of strong patent protection and effective antitrust policy. Since companies generally approach domestic markets first, final market competition and regulation is extremely important to provide incentives for capital accumulation and R&D undertakings.

All in all, U.S. institutions, and more generally, U.S. cultural attitudes (Phelps, 2003, Gordon, 2004) have been more favorable to the kind of Schumpeterian "creative destruction" that plays a key role in pharmaceutical innovation as well as in the creation and diffusion of General Purpose Technologies (Aghion and Howitt 1998b; Helpman and Trajtenberg 1998) and through it, results in higher long-term economic growth (Aghion and Griffith, 2005).

Chapter III
Main Structural Indicators

Chapter III
Main Structural Indicators

Main Findings

- Europe lags behind the U.S. in terms of pharmaceutical market size and production growth as well as internationalization through foreign direct investment (FDI) and market penetration.

- The worldwide pharmaceutical market totals €482.8 billion. Data show that from 1995 to 2005 the North American market has been growing at the highest average annual rate among OECD countries (12.3 percent), thus reaching one half of the total world market for pharmaceuticals (versus 31.2 percent in 1995).

- On the international scene, European exports largely exceed imports (more than double) resulting in a growing EU-15 sectoral trade surplus, valued at €26.953 billion in 2004. Within Europe, small countries such as Ireland, the Netherlands, Belgium, the Czech Republic and the Baltic countries are exceptionally open to trade. Overall, the U.S. is the main source and destination of extra-EU-15 trade. Japan is characterized by a consistently negative trade balance.

- Since 2002, the U.S. economy has been more open than a benchmark gravity model would predict.[1] The same conclusion can be drawn for small export-led high-growth EU countries. The opposite holds for Greece, Italy, Portugal, and Spain, possibly due to low price levels and propensity to parallel trade.[2] Moreover, a sizable growth potential emerges for the new EU member states as well as Japan, India and China.

- The capability of U.S. multinationals to access foreign markets is higher than that of their European competitors, thus EU

---

[1] The so-called gravity equation of trade predicts that the volume of trade between two countries is proportional to the size of their economy and inversely related to trade barriers between them.

[2] On this issue, see Danzon (1998) and Danzon-Chao (2000).

companies are losing ground in terms of global penetration. Foreign trade agreements have a positive effect on intra-regional pharmaceutical trade, while they do not favor regional multinationals in expanding their sales abroad.

• U.S. foreign direct investment in Europe increasingly affects the volume and direction of European international trade in pharmaceuticals especially as far as the lopsided U.S.-EU trade balance is concerned. This phenomenon is analogous in nature to the growing U.S. trade imbalance with China in manufacturing, and fuels similar, albeit sector-specific, trade tensions. This analogy deserves the utmost attention in the analysis of EU foreign trade policy to understand if and when China will attract U.S. FDI in the pharmaceutical sector away from Europe.

• The growing trade deficit of the U.S. with Europe is driven by the sharp increase of the import of pharmaceutical products from EU-based U.S. affiliates located in Europe, particularly from Ireland, and outsourcing through contract manufacturing.

• Positive growth performances of Ireland, Hungary, Sweden, and the UK are propelled by FDI, mainly from the U.S. In these countries, affiliates under foreign control account for more than 80 percent of total turnover in pharmaceuticals.[3]

• Overall, we observe vertical "resource seeking" FDI of U.S. companies in Europe, where they can replicate productivity conditions as in their home country (specifically, high capital/labor ratio and high labor productivity) but with lower costs for production factors (tax breaks, low-interest loans, low labor cost, discounts on land purchases, and government-provided infrastructure enhancements; see also Chapter II). In contrast, European investments in the U.S. are horizontal "market seeking" investments and/or vertical "knowledge seeking" investments to get access to either the U.S. final market or the U.S. market for technologies.

---

[3] In case of missing data (Ireland, Hungary) the chemical industry is considered.

- The size of the U.S. domestic market is not the only source of U.S. competitiveness. The benefits of internal market size decrease with the extent of the international integration of pharmaceutical markets. Actually, trade openness has increased over time, and as the world pharmaceutical market becomes more integrated, the benefits of large countries tend to vanish in favor of smaller countries. On the one hand, this effect can explain the positive growth performances of small northern EU countries in this sector. On the other hand, as globalization reduces the advantages of sizable internal markets, European states might have lower incentives to administrative and regulatory integration and EU pharmaceutical markets tend to be more fragmented. This is the reason why centrifugal forces have to be counterbalanced by reinvigorating the process of European pharmaceutical market integration.

III.1 Overview

In 2003, total expenditure in pharmaceuticals ranged between 0.7 percent (Luxembourg) and 2.3 percent (Slovak Republic) of GDP across OECD countries, with an average of approximately 1.5 percent.[3] The U.S. share (1.9 percent) was higher than the OECD average, whereas the EU-15 (1.4 percent) was slightly below the OECD level. The worldwide market for pharmaceuticals has doubled its size since 1995, totalling €482.8 billion in 2005.

At the end of the 1980s the pharmaceutical market was evenly distributed among North America, Europe, and the rest of the world (Africa, Asia, and Australasia—A/A/A). Since then, North America (mostly the U.S.) has significantly increased its share of total world sales, up to 44 percent in 2005, while the European market share has experienced a sharp decline in the period 2000-2002. The share of A/A/A market shrank significantly, even though it started increasing again in 2005. Short-term analyses highlight that, since 2002, North American market share has started to decrease, while Europe's has grown, except for the last year. However, the U.S. market remains by far the largest national pharmaceutical market, and is currently twice

---

[4] Source: OECD (2005a).

Table III.1   Global pharmaceutical sales and regional shares, 1989-2005 (€ billions)

Markets	'89	'90	'95	'96	'97	'98	'99	'00	'01	'02	'03	'04	'05	Average '90-'05
World market	139.1	130.2	214.3	229	261.1	268.1	312.1	386.9	434.8	449.2	434.8	442.2	482.8	—
AGR (%)	—	-6.4	64.6	6.9	14.0	2.7	16.4	24.0	12.4	3.3	-3.2	1.7	9.2	8.5
North America	34	32.4	31.2	33	35.9	39.2	41.5	44	47.2	48.4	46.7	47.8	44.2	—
AGR (%)	—	-10.8	—	13	24	12.1	23.2	31.4	20.6	5.9	-6.6	4.1	1	12.3
Europe	31	26.5	29.6	30.7	28.8	28.4	26.3	23.7	24	25	27.5	29.6	28.6	—
AGR (%)	—	-20	—	10.8	7	1.3	7.8	11.7	13.8	7.6	6.5	9.5	5.5	8.1
A/A/A[1]	30	35.1	32.4	29.2	27.5	25.1	25.9	25.8	22.9	21.7	21.4	18.8	22.3	—
AGR (%)	—	9.5	—	-3.7	7.4	-6.3	20.1	23.5	-0.2	-2.1	14.1	-10.7	29.5	4.5
Latin America	5	5.9	6.8	7.1	7.8	7.4	6.2	6.5	6	4.9	4.5	3.8	4.9	—
AGR (%)	—	10.4	—	11.6	25.2	-2.6	-2.5	30	3.7	-15.6	-11.1	-14.1	40.8	5.0

AGR = Annual Growth Rate. (1) Africa, Asia, and Australasia

Source: IMS Health—World Review (various issues, original data in USD).

as large as the EU-15 aggregate (see Table III.2; Berndt, 2001). In 2004, Europe reached a regional share up to almost 30 percent, back to the 1995 value, in large part due to the growing contribution of new EU member States such as Poland, Hungary and, to a lesser extent, the Czech Republic.

In 2005, emerging markets such as China, India and Brazil in the A/A/A regions experienced higher dynamism than European and North American markets (Table II.1). However, the largest market in Asia is still Japan, whose share of the world market in 2005 is more than 11 percent, notwithstanding a slight decline in the last few years (see Table III.2).

III.2   Trade, Growth and the Size of the Market

In the second half of the 1990s, the U.S. economy experienced a gradual but steady appreciation of the real exchange rate and a deterioration of the trade balance. This trend is called "global external imbalance" and is common to the whole U.S. economy, which has accumulated about 20 percentage points of GDP of net liabilities to the rest of the world over a decade. As we have shown in the previous chapter, during the same period of time productivity accelerated, markedly accompanied by an investment boom and followed by an expansion in the consumption of pharmaceuticals and a deterioration of the pharmaceutical trade balance. As for the trade imbalance, the productivity shock in the second half of the 1990s was also common to the whole manufacturing sector of the U.S. economy, which experienced an acceleration of TFP growth ranging from 0.5 to 2.3 percentage points (Jorgenson, 2001; Oliner e Sichel, 2000; Nordhaus, 2001; Gordon, 2002, 2003). Notably, this acceleration was specific to the U.S. economy, with little or no spillovers to other regions, and Europe was left behind (Phelps 2003; Gordon 2004).

As was argued at the end of the previous chapter, the underlying causes of the productivity gap between the U.S. and the European Union remain partially obscure and have to do with the broad U.S. institutional settings in the markets of production factors, innovation system and markets for technologies (see Chapter IV) as well as in the distribution and final market settings (see Chapter V). On the contrary, the link between U.S. productivity growth and trade imbalance has been largely documented. Using data from 1985 to 2001, Alquist and Chinn (2002) estimate that a one percentage point growth in the U.S.-EU labor productivity differential results in between a four to five percent real appreciation in the dollar/euro exchange rate. This result is somehow at odds with the well-known Harrod-Balassa-Samuelson hypothesis, according to which the real exchange rates does not respond to productivity differentials across borders but to differences in the productivity gap between sectors producing tradable and non-tradable goods. Contrary to the common wisdom, Corsetti *et al.* (2006) show that the productivity growth differentials in favor of the U.S. tend to raise U.S. output, consumption and relative price of U.S exports to other OECD countries, to improve U.S. terms of trade, and to widen the trade deficit. Moreover, the results do not depend on the measures of productivity (TFP or labor productivity, see Chapter II).

The two main reasons for the worsening of the trade balance focus on quality enhancing technological change and offshoring. The first explanation stresses the fact that productivity growth can translate into product innovation and vertical product differentiation rather

Table III.2   The size and the annual growth rate (G) of main national pharmaceutical markets (growth rates are calculated in national currencies)[1]

rank 2005		1999		2000		2001		2002		2003		2004		2005
		€ mil	G	€ mil	G	€ mil	G	€ mil	G	€ mil	G	€ mil	G	€ mil	G
1	U.S.	124,261	18	163,439	14	197,351	17	208,970	12	194,061	11	192,923	8	202,735	5
–	EU-15	72,094	8	79,962	10	90,100	10[2]	96,825	8	103,142[3]	8	111,681	–	117,149	5
2	Japan	50,246	7	62,606	3	59,744	4	55,736	1	52,092	3	52,948	1	54,450	7
3	Germany	17,135	5	18,112	6	19,904	10	21,445	8	23,288	8	23,628	2	25,616	9
4	France	16,574	5	18,066	9	19,402	7	20,117	4	21,352	6	22,878	7	24,353	6
5	Italy	10,445	8	11,961	15	13,430	12	14,089	5	14,742	4	15,490	5	15,912	3
6	UK	10,434	11	12,091	7	13,148	11	14,446	11	14,528	11	16,224	8	15,636	-2
7	Spain	6,556	16	7,692	16	8,342	10	9,144	10	10,205	12	11,260	8	12,170	8
8	Canada	5,274	11	6,843	13	7,899	17	8,476	15	8,827	11	8,828	14	10,861	7
9	China	4,290	–	5,442	–	6,316	–	6,460	8	6,576	22,	7,605	28	9,347	20
10	Brazil	5,882	–	7,243	–	6,015	–	5,318	-7	4,782	8	5,282	21	7,313	38
11	Mexico	4,440	–	6,247	–	7,318	–	7,589	13	6,450	–	6,047	9	7,075	12
15	India	3,243	9	3,706	3	4,080	12	4,152	11	3,929	8	4,561	7	5,086	9

16	Belgium	2,530	8	2,715	7	2,860	6	3,039	7	3,329	10	3,642	7	3,778	4
17	Poland	2,128	16	2,744	22	3,249	8	3,205	4	3,174	13	2,749	1	3,734	7
18	Greece	1,324	20	1,519	19	1,803	20	2,274	26	2,740	21	3,144	22	3,538	12
19	Netherlands	–	–	–	–	2,983	–	3,268	10	3,550	9	3,447	-3	3,469	1
20	Portugal	1,571	13	1,698	8	1,847	9	1,991	8	2,064	4	2,886	10	3,113	8
22	Switzerland	1,711	10	1,905	8	2,169	10	2,389	7	2,519	10	2,423	6	3,006	3
23	Sweden	2,017	11	2,327	11	2,276	7	2,474	8	2,532	2	2,618	2	2,641	4
25	Austria	1,669	11	1,762	6	1,862	6	2,032	9	2,160	6	2,312	7	2,409	4
28	Hungary	767	19	840	13	1,016	19	1,275	19	1,440	18	1,534	6	1,841	17
31	Finland	974	9	1,069	10	1,200	12	1,326	11	1,410	6	1,560	8	1,674	7
33	South Africa	898	15	1,097	19	1,027	12	901	13	1,175	12	1,478	4	1,581	5
34	Czech Republic	690	5	793	11	878	6	1,059	9	1,139	11	1,206	–	1,489	–
35	Denmark	865	8	952	10	1,044	10	1,180	13	1,243	5	1,303	–	1,414	–
38	Norway	766	13	854	9	961	11	1,180	14	1,142	3	1,137	–	1,261	–

(1) Percentage increments are rounded to integers directly in the source. (2) Cleaning of the data for Netherlands. (3) Does not include Luxembourg.
Source: IMS Health—World Review (various issues, original data in USD).
Source: IMS Health—World Review (various issues, original data in USD).Source: IMS Health—World Review (various issues, original data in USD).

than process innovation. In this case, the prices of final goods increase and productivity gains do not necessarily imply a decrease of relative price of the exports to other countries. In the next two chapters we shall demonstrate that this is often the case in pharmaceuticals.

The second explanation has to do with international division of labor, unbundling and offshoring. Starting from the beginning of the 1990s, most pharmaceutical companies have increasingly outsourced the production of bulk active ingredients and chemical intermediates (USITC, 1999). Global trade in the pharmaceutical industry has accelerated since 1995, following the elimination of duties on most medicinal chemical products under the Uruguay Round Agreement. In addition, the recent wave of mergers and acquisitions has endowed all major pharmaceutical companies of production facilities through-out the world.

Table III.3 shows pharmaceutical trade flows among the EU, the U.S., and Japan. Trade in pharmaceutical products has been increasing at higher rates in both the EU and in the U.S than in Japan. Europe has an increasingly positive trade balance, while the U.S. trade balance turned negative in 2002, mainly caused by U.S. dollar depreciation and flows of re-import from European affiliates of U.S. multinationals. While in the European case FDI and trade are complements, in Japan they are substitutes: Japan has suffered a constantly negative trade balance over the years probably due to barriers to FDI. Finally, a progressively larger share of total EU trade is made of intra-EU trade. Within Europe, import flows are unevenly distributed in favor of two major players, Germany and Ireland, which account for more than one half of the regional trade flows.

The share of EU-15 exports in pharmaceuticals towards the U.S. has increased in recent years, to the extent that the U.S. has become the main destination of EU pharmaceutical exports. Since 2002, the major exporting country to the U.S. market has been Ireland, followed by Germany and then the United Kingdom: between 2000 and 2001 there was a huge increase of imports from Ireland, making this the third largest U.S. trading partner in pharmaceuticals at that time. This is to a large extent due to intra-firm trade, i.e. re-imports from U.S. affiliates based in this country (see Table A.III.6 and Appendix III.2). The share of pharmaceutical imports to the EU from the U.S. has increased over time, reaching 55.9 percent of total EU imports in

2004. The main destinations are the Netherlands, United Kingdom, France and Germany. In particular, in 2004, exports towards Netherlands almost doubled with respect to 2003, whereas flows to other countries remained almost stable.

Not only is the U.S. by far the largest national pharmaceutical market (see Table III.2), it has also grown rapidly in the last decade. Alongside this, the U.S. outperforms Europe and Japan in pharmaceuticals both in terms of growth of drug production, as well as in terms of its share of all-manufacturing production (see Table II.2). Figure III.1 shows that the value of pharmaceutical production is highly related to the size of domestic markets.

The literature on the relationship between market size, trade, and growth is vast and a comprehensive survey is well beyond the scope of this work. Nonetheless, from Adam Smith's contribution on the relationship between the size of the market and division of labor[5] to recent contributions on increasing returns and endogenous technological change,[6] economists have identified the positive correlation between the size of the market and productivity gains and competitiveness.

In particular, it is well-known that home-demand conditions can help to build and sustain competitive advantage in industries characterized by a vibrant domestic market *vis-à-vis* foreign markets (Porter, 1985). The nature and the intensity of product market competition is more important than size *per se* (Aghion and Howitt, 1998a). National companies gain competitive advantage if domestic buyers are the world most advanced and demanding buyers. Home demand can help domestic companies gain global competitive advantages if their needs anticipate or even shape those of other nations. Thus, domestic market size and demand conditions are well-known determinants of international competitiveness and attractiveness (Linder, 1961, Vernon, 1966).

However, as Alesina *et al.* (2003) have pointed out, the market size accessible to a country's domestic industry will only coincide with a country market in an autarkic economy. On the contrary, the size of

---

[5] Smith (1776).
[6] See Romer (1986), Lucas (1988) and Grossman and Helpman (1991).

Table III.3   International trade in pharmaceutical products (€ millions)

	1991	1992	1993	1994	1995	1996	1997	1998	1999	2000	2001	2002	2003	2004
EU exports														
intra EU-15	12,150	13,785	14,513	17,128	19,736	21,017	24,392	28,225	32,918	38,993	47,849	72,142	74,410	81,978
extra EU-15	10,324	11,583	14,016	15,318	17,207	19,161	24,020	27,517	32,296	39,731	47,036	54,024	55,457	56,927
EU-10	430	544	800	1,062	1,269	1,532	1,980	2,321	2,477	2,976	3,639	4,009	4,250	4,691
U.S.	1,604	1,894	2,247	2,425	2,692	3,715	5,043	6,771	8,907	11,045	14,541	19,528	20,528	21,152
Switzerland	932	1,163	1,477	1,562	1,884	1,972	2,526	2,987	3,758	4,583	6,232	7,457	7,427	7,841
Japan	1,418	1,733	2,043	2,214	2,337	2,146	2,243	1,880	2,567	3,224	3,467	3,500	3,263	3,468
Canada	292	311	385	408	437	479	635	779	966	1,331	1,886	2,163	2,475	2,668
Rest of world	5,647	5,938	7,063	7,648	8,589	9,318	11,593	12,779	13,621	16,572	17,271	17,367	17,514	17,109
Total	22,473	25,368	28,528	32,446	36,944	40,178	48,412	55,742	65,214	78,724	94,884	126,165	129,868	138,905
EU imports														
Intra EU-15	12,150	13,785	14,513	17,128	19,736	21,017	24,392	28,225	32,918	38,993	47,849	72,142	74,410	81,978
Extra EU-15	5,120	5,881	6,812	7,386	8,452	9,689	11,076	12,878	14,995	17,928	22,860	24,963	25,312	29,974
Total	17,270	19,666	21,325	24,515	28,189	30,706	35,468	41,103	47,913	56,920	70,709	97,105	99,723	111,953
Trade balance Extra EU-15	5,203	5,702	7,203	7,932	8,755	9,472	12,944	14,640	17,302	21,804	24,176	29,061	30,145	26,953
Trade balance EU-15-U.S.	-52	15	-34	-48	-228	-120	299	775	1,651	1,645	1,617	5,649	6,363	4,383
U.S. exports														
EU-25	1,668	1,905	2,326	2,530	2,995	3,936	4,890	6,155	7,453	9,652	13,266	14,246	14,553	17,048
EU-15	1,656	1,879	2,281	2,473	2,919	3,835	4,744	5,996	7,256	9,401	12,925	13,879	14,165	16,769
EU-10	13	26	45	56	75	101	146	159	197	252	341	367	387	279

	1991	1992	1993	1994	1995	1996	1997	1998	1999	2000	2001	2002	2003	2004
Switzerland	86	122	244	410	243	217	484	454	803	919	1,199	1,028	890	1,094
Japan	672	658	830	792	849	821	895	885	1,045	1,175	1,357	1,366	1,208	1,214
Canada	430	564	744	771	745	880	1,152	1,360	1,750	2,387	2,445	2,514	2,529	2,421
Rest of the world	937	1,083	1,211	1,287	1,314	1,706	2,075	2,412	2,893	3,369	4,064	3,770	3,596	3,592
Total	3,793	4,332	5,356	5,789	6,146	7,560	9,497	11,266	13,943	17,503	22,330	22,923	22,775	25,368
U.S. imports														
Total	2,494	2,972	3,573	3,982	4,283	5,629	7,775	9,794	12,805	16,079	20,939	26,305	28,058	28,436
Trade Balance U.S.	1,300	1,360	1,783	1,807	1,863	1,931	1,722	1,473	1,138	1,424	1,391	-3,381	-5,283	-3,068
Japan exports														
EU-25	340	451	529	557	674	723	794	737	883	1,057	1,224	1,169	1,243	1,333
EU-15	*337*	*448*	*523*	*549*	*667*	*712*	*781*	*719*	*859*	*1,029*	*1,189*	*1,128*	*1,204*	*1,308*
EU-10	*3*	*3*	*6*	*8*	*8*	*11*	*13*	*18*	*24*	*28*	*36*	*41*	*39*	*26*
Switzerland	9	7	21	14	16	23	32	35	45	62	103	110	102	126
U.S.	220	254	342	385	402	499	640	803	1,235	1,665	1,806	1,985	2,130	1,814
Canada	6	8	16	24	25	31	31	29	30	19	15	27	26	44
Rest of world	396	412	477	474	497	517	577	530	630	735	717	684	641	632
Total	971	1,132	1,385	1,455	1,614	1,793	2,074	2,134	2,823	3,538	3,866	3,976	4,142	3,950
Japan imports														
Total	2,512	2,828	3,355	3,548	3,758	3,544	3,740	3,344	4,309	5,168	5,640	5,738	5,475	5,719
Trade Balance Japan	-1,541	-1,696	-1,970	-2,093	-2,143	-1,751	-1,667	-1,210	-1,486	-1,630	-1,774	-1,762	-1,333	-1,769

Our calculation based on the NBER-UN World Trade (1986-2000) and UN Comtrade (2001-2004).
Data for exports are based on imports of partner countries to achieve consistency.

Table III.4   EU-15 imports from member countries in pharmaceutical products (€ millions and share of total imports)

Countries	2000		2001		2002		2003		2004	
	value	%	value	%	value	%	value	%	value	%
Austria	656.74	1.7	855.09	1.8	1,060.54	1.5	1,012.54	1.4	1,117.85	1.5
Belgium	2,884.12	7.6	3,571.39	7.5	4,468.14	6.2	5,109.11	6.9	6,243.97	8.2
Denmark	1,665.88	4.4	2,073.45	4.3	2,506.70	3.5	2,309.84	3.1	2,087.49	2.7
Finland	148.03	0.4	197.14	0.4	226.50	0.3	203.89	0.3	234.96	0.3
France	5,725.70	15.0	7,082.93	14.8	7,647.36	10.6	8,228.61	11.1	8,449.82	11.1
Germany	6,241.55	16.4	7,489.91	15.7	13,167.05	18.3	15,646.82	21.0	18,251.65	24.0
Greece	197.42	0.5	317.37	0.7	437.39	0.6	458.95	0.6	582.41	0.8
Ireland	3,917.73	10.3	5,446.10	11.4	20,384.13	28.3	18,420.57	24.8	20,162.26	26.5
Italy	3,683.11	9.7	4,786.21	10.0	3,968.93	5.5	4,135.90	5.6	4,824.26	6.3
Luxembourg	146.34	0.4	283.89	0.6	511.91	0.7	343.24	0.5	349.70	0.5
Netherlands	3,130.97	8.2	3,611.70	7.6	4,125.13	5.7	4,109.87	5.5	4,488.29	5.9
Portugal	148.88	0.4	194.25	0.4	188.34	0.3	178.81	0.2	191.11	0.3
Spain	1,656.73	4.3	2,149.58	4.5	2,737.20	3.8	2,969.74	4.0	3,159.09	4.1
Sweden	2,396.06	6.3	2,711.68	5.7	2,823.82	3.9	3,079.11	4.1	2,700.05	3.5
UK	5,527.19	14.5	7,040.00	14.7	7,851.53	10.9	8,166.08	11.0	3,358.69	4.4

Source: UN Comtrade

the accessible market is independent from a country market size in the case of frictionless international trade.

Therefore, assuming absent barriers to trade, internal market size becomes irrelevant for competitiveness. However, a vast literature has persuasively demonstrated that even in the absence of explicit trade barriers, nations appear to trade too much with themselves and too little with each other (McCallum, 1995; Trefler, 1995; Helliwell, 1998, Eaton and Kortum, 2000).

Indeed, the size of the market depends on both domestic demand and trade openness, while the relationship between market size and industrial competitiveness is mediated by the trade regime. In a regime of free trade, small countries can succeed, while in the presence of significant trade barriers, the size of the internal market is much more important for growth and competitiveness.

Table III.6 shows that from 1995 to 2003 the index of trade openness has been increasing in most countries. The trade openness ratio

Table III.5 Trade flows between the U.S. and EU-15 countries in pharmaceutical products (€ millions)

	U.S. Imports					U.S. Exports				
	2000	2001	2002	2003	2004	2000	2001	2002	2003	2004
Austria	298.3	376.2	643.8	569.5	452.2	127.9	174.1	211.5	136.5	127.2
Belgium	552.2	740.1	698.4	706.2	626.3	1,007.9	1,061.4	1,646.5	1,644.9	1,578.9
Denmark	256.1	427.8	563.6	626.5	685.7	20.9	37.4	38.2	53.8	101.5
Finland	33.0	87.7	97.3	125.3	109.4	12.9	16.7	8.9	10.4	17.4
France	1,105.6	1,904.8	2,280.6	2,532.3	2,927.0	1,205.6	1,599.6	1,694.6	1,591.5	1,791.5
Germany	2,487.5	2,832.3	3,392.7	3,595.1	4,129.8	704.1	937.8	709.2	1,003.3	1,575.2
Greece	0.0	0.0	0.0	0.0	0.1	30.8	36.2	25.6	23.8	79.9
Ireland	758.9	2.427.7	5.674.9	4.972.2	4.729.1	416.2	527.7	518.1	493.5	519.1
Italy	1.435.7	979.4	786.5	775.8	897.4	1.011.0	844.7	836.5	869.7	776.9
Luxembourg	0.0	0.0	0.1	0.0	0.0	2.3	0.3	0.0	0.1	0.1
Netherlands	330.8	471.7	446.1	336.8	348.9	650.5	969.2	1,430.2	1,725.3	2,855.5
Portugal	29.6	29.2	33.7	38.6	27.6	10.2	11.3	9.8	7.9	9.5
Spain	52.2	65.0	173.6	277.2	364.8	217.8	290.4	212.1	240.8	379.8
Sweden	769.8	706.2	848.0	1,417.0	1,782.8	116.9	91.4	128.5	114.9	93.1
UK	2,937.3	3,493.3	3,888.4	4,555.7	4,070.3	1,547.6	2,868.4	2,008.5	1,695.5	1,845.4

Source: UN Comtrade

(TOR) is computed by dividing the average of imports and exports by value added. In 2000, EU-15 TOR was much higher than in the United States. Japan presented the lowest value of the index among the countries considered.

Within Europe, it is not surprising that small countries such as Ireland, Belgium, the Netherlands, the Czech Republic and the Baltic countries are exceptionally open to trade. Among them, Ireland and Belgium have significantly increased the value of their TOR in 2003. On the contrary, Sweden and Denmark, together with Poland, Hungary, and Slovenia experienced a fall in the value of the index in 2003.

The total extent of the market given by both domestic demand and trade openness, can partially explain the high growth performances of both the U.S. and small EU countries.

Nevertheless, barriers and frictions to trade, cross-border circulation of technological competences and factors of production still pres-

Figure III.1   Pharmaceutical market size versus total production, (€), double logarithmic scale, 2003

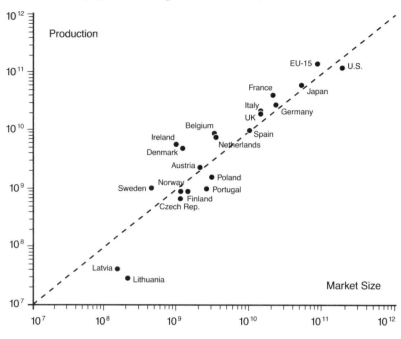

(1) The EU-15 data point refers to 2001.

ent in EU,[7] confer to U.S. companies a significant advantage. Hence, the need to give priority to the administrative and regulatory integration of the European pharmaceutical market to enhance the competitiveness of the European drug industry.

III.3   Size, Barriers and "the Mystery of Missing Trade"

In this section, we analyze world trade data to evaluate countries' performance, once the potential determinants of international trade, most notably market size, internal production and geographical distance, have been taken into account.

---

[7] The formation of a single market for pharmaceuticals in Europe has achieved some progress, especially in the field of market approval, through the establishment of EMEA (European Medicines Evaluation Agency), which can release market authorizations valid throughout EU. However, the differences in price regulation mechanisms and industrial policies among Member States still contribute to a fragmented structure. Barriers to market integration arise from different brand names under which the same products are sold, as well as from the dissimilar pricing and reimbursement schemes provided in each EU country (Kanavos, 1998).

Table III.6   Trade openness ratio (TOR), values and growth rates (%), 1995-2003

	1995	2000		2003	
	TOR	TOR	%	TOR	%
U.S.	0.12	0.19	*58.43*	0.26	*36.75*
Japan	0.10	0.13	*28.05*	0.17	*30.78*
EU-15	—	0.59	—	—	—
Germany	—	1.48	—	2.10	*41.84*
France	0.67[1]	1.02	*51.17*	1.22	*20.14*
UK	1.01[1]	1.26	*24.35*	1.86	*47.13*
Italy	0.69	1.12	*60.97*	1.33	*19.28*
Spain	0.60	1.21	*102.17*	1.86	*53.16*
Belgium	1.60	2.11	*32.01*	4.23	*100.03*
Netherlands	2.36	3.30	*39.98*	4.91	*48.89*
Sweden	1.09	1.18	*7.83*	0.93[2]	*-21.40*
Ireland	1.42	1.51	*6.88*	5.07[2]	*235.45*
Denmark	1.30	1.43	*10.07*	1.37	*-4.32*
Austria	1.89	1.90	*0.45*	2.45	*29.29*
Poland	1.32[1]	1.66	*25.64*	1.44[2]	*-13.38*
Hungary	1.04[3]	1.13	*8.69*	1.04	*-8.24*
Portugal	1.02[1]	1.94	*89.17*	2.40	*23.62*
Finland	0.99	1.45	*46.58*	2.08	*44.16*
Norway	1.19[1]	1.51	*27.14*	1.65	*9.21*
Slovenia	1.16	1.48	*28.32*	0.93	*-36.96*
Czech Republic	—	3.05	—	3.07	*0.76*
Slovakia	2.20	5.07	*130.22*	7.14	*41.01*
Estonia	—	—	—	9.90	—
Latvia	1.68[4]	3.01	*79.04*	5.76	*91.15*
Lithuania	—	9.53	—	17.37[2]	*82.34*

TOR = (Exports+Imports)÷(2×Value Added)
(1) 1996; (2) 2002; (3) 1998; (4) 1997

Source: our computations on UN Comtrade

Trade is positively related to the size of the economic partners and is limited by their distance due to increases in transaction costs (e.g. transport costs). Ceteris paribus, a high level of production of a given economy increases the availability of goods and services for exports, while a high income determines a higher demand for foreign products and therefore higher imports.

Gravity Models

Gravity models are popular tools for statistical analyses of bilateral flows between different geographical entities. The basic model was first proposed by Tinbergen (1962). In their simplest form gravity models state that the volume of trade between any two countries is positively related to the size of their economies and inversely related to the trade costs between them. Thus, larger countries tend to trade more with each other. These models perform extremely well empirically. However, despite its remarkable explanatory capacity, the gravity equation was until very recently criticized for lacking a theoretical foundation. For this reason it was almost completely abandoned till the late 1980s.

In the meantime, theoretical foundations have been proposed adding more realistic specifications than those found in the early literature, including product differentiation (Anderson 1979) and monopolistic competition (Bergstrand, 1985, 1989).

In this setting, trading countries produce differentiated goods sold in the international markets. In a monopolistic competition model with open economies trading freely, countries are specialized in producing different qualities of the same products, and hence they simply export to each other different varieties (intra industry trade).

Since the 1990s the gravity trade model has regained interest. Gravity models have been used to analyze a wide set of trade questions of direct concern to policy-makers. For instance, most studies have extensively employed these tools to assess the ex-post trade effects of regional trade agreements (see, for example, Frankel-Rose, 2000). Furthermore, recent developments of theories modeling multinationals' strategies have encouraged the use of gravity models to explore how foreign direct investment into regionally integrated areas impacts on trade flows.

In this context, we explore trade flows in the pharmaceutical sector. The gravity model allows us to net out the "obvious" effects of size and distance from trade flows and to evaluate a country performance in international trade.

Analytically, the simplest form of the gravity model is the following:

$$F_{ij} = G_j \frac{M_i M_j}{D_{ij}^2} \quad [\text{eq. } 1]$$

where F_{ij} usually is the export flows from country i to country j (or bilateral flow between the two countries); M_i and M_j proxy the economic size of exporting and importing geographical entities; D_{ij} represents the distance between the two locations; G_j is a sort of remoteness measure for the importing country. The rationale of this variable is that countries with many nearby sources of goods, i.e. with lower value of G, will import less from each particular source.

Using logarithms, equation 1 can be expressed in linear form:

$$\ln(F_{ij}) = \alpha + \beta \ln(M_i) + \gamma \ln(M_j) - \theta \ln(D_{ij}) \quad [\text{eq. } 2]$$

The "theoretical" values predicted for the gravity equation are $\beta = \gamma = 1$ and $\theta = 2$. This means that bilateral trade flows are directly proportional to the two countries' economic size, while distance affects more than proportional exports from country i to country j.

In the following, we estimate a gravity model for trade in pharmaceuticals and analyze for each country, the differences of the estimated coefficients from the theoretical values suggested by the literature (see box "Gravity Models"). The same model is estimated for total manufacturing (excluding pharmaceuticals). Differences in the estimated coefficients of the two equations allow us to understand better the characteristics of international trade in pharmaceuticals, disentangling the industry's specific features from general trends. Furthermore, through the analysis of the residuals, we detect countries' deviations from the theoretical model, in order to find whether there is some competitive advantage or disadvantage implied in trade flows pattern for each country.

Data on trade flows in pharmaceuticals and total manufactured goods are drawn from the NBER-UN World Trade Database (Feenstra *et al.*, 2005) and from the UN Comtrade Database. Additional data used in the gravity model come from various sources including: Eurostat, OECD-STAN Database, UNIDO, the Chinese Statistical Office, the World Bank, and IMS Health Data. As a whole, we considered the EU-25 countries, the OECD countries outside the EU, China, and India.

Table III.7 reports estimation results on a cross-section dataset referred to the year 2000. In the analysis of the pharmaceutical industry, the variables included in the gravity equation are production of the exporting country and market size of the importing country, whereas in the case of total manufacturing we consider gross production value and final consumption expenditure. In the baseline specification of the model (1) only the economic masses of the countries involved in the transaction are considered. In the second version of the model (2), we add the distance between the countries[8] among the regressors. In Models (3) and (4) dummies account for contiguous countries and Free Trade Associations (FTAs). Namely, we consider NAFTA, EU-15, and the new EU member states as regional blocs.

In all the different specifications, the main theoretical predictions of the gravity model are confirmed. As expected, production and market size have a positive and significant effect on trade flows, while geographical distance exerts a negative effect.

Estimated coefficients of the production and market variables are consistent with the theoretical values provided for the Gravity Model. The coefficient for distance is lower for pharmaceuticals than for total manufacturing, implying a lower effect of distance on pharmaceutical product flows with respect to other products. Coherently, the contiguous country dummy (equal to one if countries share their borders) significantly increases the total manufacturing[9] trade, whereas it does not affect pharmaceutical products' international trade. Regional trade integration (Free Trade Association, i.e. FTA in Model 3) has a positive and significant impact on export flows, but a higher effect is estimated in the case of trade in pharmaceuticals.

---

[8] According to the main recent literature, geographical distance has been calculated following the great circle formula, which uses latitudes and longitudes of the most important cities in terms of population (for survey of the empirical evidence on international trade, see Leamer and Levinsohn, 1994).

[9] Pharmaceutical products are excluded.

**Table III.7   Trade in pharmaceutical products:
gravity model estimates**

Variable	(1) Pharma	(1) TotMnf (excl. Pharma)[1]	(2) Pharma	(2) TotMnf (excl. Pharma)	(3) Pharma	(3) TotMnf (excl. Pharma)	(4) Pharma	(4) TotMnf (excl. Pharma)
Production	0.807	0.842	0.961	1.049	0.937	1.031	0.948	1.041
	0.031	*0.030*	*0.029*	*0.019*	*0.028*	*0.019*	*0.030*	*0.020*
Market	0.550	0.673	0.705	0.854	0.673	0.835	0.688	0.847
	0.039	*0.030*	*0.034*	*0.019*	*0.032*	*0.019*	*0.034*	*0.020*
Distance	–	–	-0.873	-0.982	-0.639	-0.868	-0.634	-0.880
	–	–	*0.047*	*0.028*	*0.058*	*0.0360*	*0.058*	*0.036*
Cont.C.	–	–	–	–	0.053	0.463	0.106	0.394
	–	–	–	–	*0.196*	*0.120*	*0.201*	*0.124*
FTA	–	–	–	–	1.074	0.244	–	–
	–	–	–	–	*0.121*	*0.074*	–	–
NAFTA	–	–	–	–	–	–	-0.170	0.622*
	–	–	–	–	–	–	*0.550*	*0.337*
EU-15	–	–	–	–	–	–	1.076	0.181
	–	–	–	–	–	–	*0.128*	*0.079*
NMS	–	–	–	–	–	–	1.299	0.503
	–	–	–	–	–	–	*0.256*	*0.158*
Cons.	-13.280	-19.027	-13.203	-21.402	-14.116	-21.425	-14.752	-21.910
	1.153	*1.160*	*0.955*	*0.694*	*0.915*	*0.685*	*0.996*	*0.759*
N	749	748	749	748	749	748	749	748
R squared	0.497	0.627	0.657	0.858	0.689	0.863	0.691	0.864

(1) Total manufacturing other than pharmaceuticals.

Source: our computation on data from Eurostat, OECD (The STAN Database), UNIDO, the Chinese Statistical Office, the World Bank, IMS Health Data, NBER World Trade Database, CEPII.

There are some differences among regional trade blocs. In particular, the EU pharmaceutical industry is characterized by higher levels of market integration than free trade areas such as the NAFTA, which has a positive impact on total manufacturing but not on pharmaceuticals. This is likely due to the different characteristics of trading partners on the two sides of the Ocean. Indeed, U.S. exports in the drug industry are mainly directed towards extra-regional markets (see Table III.3).

All econometric specifications, estimated coefficients for pharmaceuticals are smaller than for total manufacturing.

The inspection of residuals sheds light onto country-specific deviations from the prediction of a pure gravity law of trade. Figure III.2 shows the average residuals, when the country acts as an importer and as an exporter. The fitted values have been obtained using coefficient estimates of regression in Model (4) of Table III.7. Positive residuals indicate that the country has a trade performance that is higher than the one predicted by the theoretical model, therefore having some source of competitive advantage. The reverse is true for negative residuals: the country has a flow of products which is lower than the one predicted by the model, therefore not being outward oriented (negative exporter residuals) or having some institutional setting that design a less attractive market (negative importer residuals).

Residuals have been standardized to compare the deviations of the pharmaceutical industry gravity model with the deviations of the analogous regression of total manufacturing (net of pharmaceuticals).

Considering import flows, the U.S. turns out to be more open than predicted by the gravity model. This finding is mostly due to re-imports of U.S. affiliates from abroad, i.e. intra company trade, which is particularly relevant in the drug industry. Also in the case of total manufacturing, the U.S. presents positive average residuals but the competitive advantage results are less evident than in the previous case.

Other positive deviations (greater openness) emerge for Australia, New Zealand and Switzerland. While in the case of Australia and New Zealand this outcome is the effect of remoteness and it holds for total manufacturing, Swiss import flows in pharmaceuticals are due to the presence of the headquarters of major multinational companies (MNCs), whose production plants are mostly settled abroad. However, the negative deviations are by far more interesting.

Major negative deviations are evident for Austria, Finland, Greece, Italy, Portugal, and Spain. All these are EU countries with low price and weaker patent protection, therefore foreign companies have fewer incentives to operate in these countries because of the possible negative spillovers on other EU national markets through reference pricing or parallel trade. First, prices in these countries are usually set as a benchmark to determine price at launch for drugs in other EU markets. Second, Austria, France, Greece, Italy, Portugal, and Spain have been traditionally considered as source countries of parallel traded pharmaceutical products. In these markets, the average price level is usually lower than that of potential destination countries, hence making them a potential source of parallel exports for some products (Kanavos *et al.*, 2004). As most of these countries have a negative balance in terms of licensing, we can conjecture that they perform a relatively higher percentage of total production through licensing agreements with local producers, instead of trade, nourishing a fringe of small national pharmaceutical companies (see Table IV.14 and Chapter V).

As far as export is concerned, we observe positive performances of export-led, high growth, small EU countries (Ireland, Belgium, Denmark, the Netherlands and Sweden[10]). This result is larger in pharmaceuticals than in total manufacturing, and it is probably linked to their specific capacity of attracting foreign investments in the pharmaceutical sector. In particular, market seeking FDI undertaken by U.S. firms unavoidably foster the exports of these countries (see Table III.12). The case of Ireland is particularly clear-cut and it exemplifies the extent to which foreign ownership of enterprises can affect export performance of the host countries. Thus, Ireland serves primarily as an export platform for the foreign companies that use it as a production location (see Barba Navaretti, 2004; Appendix III.2).

Negative deviations from the predictions of a gravity model are detected in the case of emerging economies. This finding is noteworthy as it is industry specific. In fact, all countries except Mexico and Poland have a positive export performance in total manufacturing. New EU member states such as Poland, Hungary, the Czech Republic and Slovenia are currently underperforming as compared to their potential in terms of pharmaceutical exports. The same is true for India and China. The case of China is particularly interesting since it still has a wide margin for growth in international trade for pharmaceutical products, even though it has already gained a large competitive advantage in terms of total manufacturing exports. This conclusion is further supported by the findings, reported in Chapter IV, of an increased effort of emerging countries in pharmaceutical research, development and production.

An analogous argument holds for Hungary, even though the difference among the average residuals between total manufacturing and

---

[10]Sweden also shows a considerable negative average residual as an importer.

pharmaceuticals is lower. This country poses itself as a potential net exporter of generic products. Top generic producers are located in this country, for example Gedeon Richter and Biogal, a subsidiary of Teva. Therefore, given the competitive advantage enjoyed in total manufacturing exports and the internal structure of its pharmaceutical market, huge potential for pharmaceutical exports is detected.

Finally, countries with stringent price controls (and negative departures in terms of imports) do not display large positive export residual departures from the model's predictions. A possible explanation is that their national companies face high costs to enter foreign markets, and because of low prices in their initial launch markets, they are not able to cover with profits the fixed costs of launch in foreign countries (Kyle, 2006). Furthermore, this result could also be explained by a different product specialization of European countries, with southern European countries specializing in low-cost/low-quality pharmaceuticals and northern European countries with a relative higher share of high-cost/high quality production over total production.

III.4   Trade, Outsourcing and Offshoring

As shown in Section III.2, the EU-15 aggregate has experienced a growing sectoral trade surplus, summing up to €26.953 billion[11] in 2004 (€4.383 billion of which with the U.S.). European exports are more than double European imports. The opposite holds for the U.S., where domestic demand exceeds local production. Thus, the U.S. has experienced a growing sectoral trade deficit, which in 2004 equals €3.068 billion (see Table III.6 and Table A.III.1).

Looking jointly at the dynamics of the U.S. trade balance, U.S. trade flows with Europe and the value of imports from U.S. affiliates in Europe, it becomes clear that, beginning in 1995, the U.S. trade imbalance in pharmaceuticals has been driven by the growing delocalization of pharmaceutical production in Europe though offshoring and outsourcing. The delocalization trend has sustained the import of drugs from European contract manufacturing organizations (CMOs) and affiliates of U.S. multinational corporations located in Europe[12] (see Figure III.3). Global trade in the pharmaceutical industry has increased

---

[11] Intra EU-15 trade is not considered.

[12] This argument is extensively developed in Chapter II.

Figure III.2   Departures from the gravity model of trade flows (import/export) in pharmaceuticals as compared to total manufacturing[1]

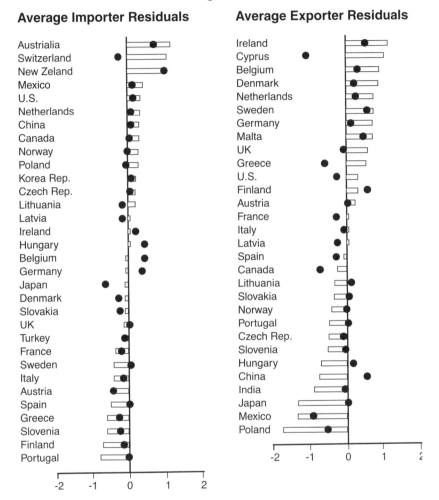

Average Importer Residuals

Austrialia
Switzerland
New Zeland
Mexico
U.S.
Netherlands
China
Canada
Norway
Poland
Korea Rep.
Czech Rep.
Lithuania
Latvia
Ireland
Hungary
Belgium
Germany
Japan
Denmark
Slovakia
UK
Turkey
France
Sweden
Italy
Austria
Spain
Greece
Slovenia
Finland
Portugal

Average Exporter Residuals

Ireland
Cyprus
Belgium
Denmark
Netherlands
Sweden
Germany
Malta
UK
Greece
U.S.
Finland
Austria
France
Italy
Latvia
Spain
Canada
Lithuania
Slovakia
Norway
Portugal
Czech Rep.
Slovenia
Hungary
China
India
Japan
Mexico
Poland

(1) Total manufacturing residuals are denoted with bullets.

since the beginning of 1995 following the elimination of duties on most medicinal chemical products under the Uruguay Round Agreement. In addition, the recent wave of mergers and acquisitions has endowed all major pharmaceutical companies of production facilities throughout the world. This is particularly evident in 2001 and 2002.

According to our computations, exchange rate fluctuations affected the trade balance only marginally. In the worst case scenario, i.e. U.S. exports denominated in U.S. dollars and U.S. imports denominated in euros, exchange rate fluctuations account for at most 27 percent of the trade imbalance in 2001-2002. As a result, in 2003 U.S. imports of medicinal chemicals accounted for about one-third of the growth in U.S. imports from the EU. Nearly one-half of U.S. imports of medicinal chemicals from the EU is composed of drugs supplied by Ireland, mostly cardiovascular drugs and active pharmaceutical ingredients (USITC, 2004). In recent years, U.S. companies have taken advantage of Ireland's national tax policy favoring research-oriented corporations, lower production costs, advanced manufacturing technology, and skilled work force to establish production facilities to supply the U.S. and European markets (see Appendix III.2).

The growing U.S. trade imbalance is not sector specific but is common to the whole U.S. economy. Overall, the U.S. good and services trade deficit reached a record level of $764 billion (6.2 percent of GDP) in 2006. Manufactured imports are responsible for the bulk of the U.S. trade deficit (82.5 percent). Offshoring, that is to say the international division of labor within MNCs, accounted for 47 percent of U.S. imports in 2005 and has grown rapidly in recent years (Grossman and Rossi-Hansberg, 2006). Since 2003, after China fully completed the harmonization of its system to the WTO and oil prices began to soar, the growth of the U.S. merchandise trade deficit has accelerated, driven largely by petroleum imports (2.2 percent of GDP) and the trade deficit with China (1.8 percent of GDP), while the residual component of the trade deficit (2.2 percent of GDP), including U.S.-EU trade, has declined. Back to pharmaceuticals, in the same period of time intra-company trade with Europe experienced a sudden reduction, U.S.-EU trade in pharmaceuticals flattered and a the intra-company trade balance with U.S. affiliates in Asia turned negative. The overall picture suggests that the U.S.-EU trade relationship is close to a turning point. U.S. multinational corporations have already outsourced part of their production capacity in Europe and are ready to relocate part of it in Singapore, Taiwan, China and India.[13]

---

[13] In February 2007, Pfizer announced the intention to significantly cut back its manufacturing capacity in Ireland as part of a plan to reduce the number of manufacturing sites from 93 to 48 by the end of 2008, while at the same time increasing its outsourcing, especially to lower cost destinations. Almost simultaneously, Pfizer announced that it had decided to outsource the manufacture of some of its active pharmaceutical ingredients (APIs) to two Asian contract manufacturers, ScinoPharm of Taiwan and Shanghai Pharmaceutical Co. of China.

Figure III.3 The U.S. trade balance in pharmaceuticals, current € billion

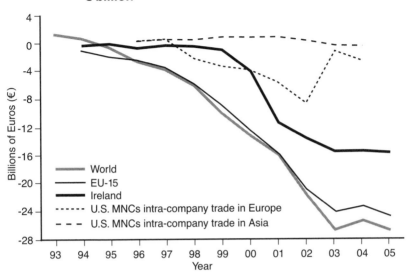

Source: BEA (2006); USITC (2005, 2001, 1998), Lenz (2000).

Table III.8 Pharmaceutical production (sales) of foreign affiliates of multinational corporations (MNCs)

Production Current € millions	PANEL A: Production by affiliates of foreign MNCs (majority owned) in the U.S.			PANEL B: Production by U.S. MNCs (majority owned) affiliates located outside the U.S.		
	Total	Europe	% of Europe on total	Total	Europe	% of Europe on total
1996	37,425	—	—	—	—	—
1997	43,092	40,353	93.6	43,512	31,300	71.9
1998	46,151	43,795	94.9	52,805	36,150	68.5
1999	47,361	45,229	95.5	54,938	39,512	71.9
2000	63,563	61,022	96.0	64,034	44,437	69.4
2001	70,338	67,006	95.3	78,969	53,745	68.1
2002	74,669	69,645	93.3	85,651	58,969	68.8
2003	68,248	64,435	94.4	97,856	71,077	72.6
2004	67,116	62,089	92.5	94,071	70,537	75.0

Source: BEA (2006)

As for the pharmaceutical trade balance, Figure III.3 shows that it turned negative in 1995, driven by the trade deficit with Europe caused by the sharp increase of the import of pharmaceutical products from European affiliates of U.S. MNCs.

By analyzing the relationship between FDI and exports in pharmaceuticals, we find a positive relationship between affiliate production and both parent country exports and industry exports (see Lipsey and Weiss, 1981 and 1984).

As we will see in the next section, U.S. multinationals have been able to successfully break through into European markets in terms of sales. However, at the same time, U.S. imports of pharmaceuticals from U.S. affiliates in Europe have soared.

Table III.8 shows that the production of the thirty-one majority-owned affiliates of foreign MNCs located in the U.S. and Europe has increased in recent years. Notably, the relationship between Europe and the U.S. strengthened: almost all the production of affiliates located in the U.S. belongs to European parents, and more than 70 percent of the production of affiliates located in Europe to U.S. parents.

If it is true that the international division of labor within MNCs accounts for a large fraction of trade flows of pharmaceuticals among industrialized countries, it is also true that U.S. enterprises lead this globalization process. Indeed, in 2004, total sales of U.S. MNCs' affiliates located outside the U.S. were 40 percent higher than the total sales of the foreign affiliates in the U.S.

Table III.9 shows that the value of U.S. pharmaceutical products imported from U.S. owned affiliates settled abroad has grown from €1.397 billion in 1996 to €7.090 billion in 2004, after a peak of €11.807 billion in 2002. During that year, U.S. exports to affiliates of U.S.-based multinationals were by far lower, amounting to €3.739 billion. However, in 2004 they increased up to €4.850 billion. Over time, a clear-cut trend emerges: in 1998 imports from U.S. affiliates started to be higher than exports, revealing a clear offshoring pattern and intra-company trade.

Thus, in 2004 the U.S. imported pharmaceuticals through foreign MNCs' affiliates for a net value of €2.240 billion after a record high of €8.068 billion in 2002.

Table III.9 The offshoring of U.S. pharmaceutical production

PANEL A: U.S. imports from MNCs affiliates located abroad (majority-owned)			
Re-imports current € millions	Total	% shipped directly to their own parents	of which European
1996	1,397	88.4	1,115
1997	1,411	85.9	1,123
1998	3,938	95.7	—
1999	5,078	98.2	4,704
2000	6,280	98.1	5,919
2001	8,526	98.2	8,069
2002	11,807	96.9	11,068
2003	6,821	96.4	5,763
2004	7,090	96.3	6,091

PANEL B: U.S. exports to MNCs affiliates abroad (majority-owned)			
Re-imports current € millions	Total	% shipped directly to their own parents	of which European
1996	2,389	92.9	1,206
1997	2,854	93.3	1,514
1998	2,893	94.1	1,549
1999	3,388	94.5	1,554
2000	3,736	90.1	1,696
2001	4,052	93.3	1,801
2002	3,739	91.3	1,809
2003	5,766	87.4	4,593
2004	4,850	95.5	4,063

Note: data for 2004 are preliminary

Source: BEA (2006)

In 2004 U.S. imports through U.S.-based affiliates of foreign MNCs were more than €10 billion, while the relative U.S. exports were about half (Table III.10).

Overall, we observe that intra-firm trade of foreign MNCs with affiliate companies in the U.S. exceeds trade of U.S. MNCs with affiliates abroad in all years with the exception of 2002. Needless to say, the European Union has a cost advantage in the production of pharmaceuticals *vis-à-vis* the U.S. Hence, manufacturing of pharmaceuticals for the U.S. market has been partially relocated from the U.S. toward some European countries, and European companies prefer to serve the U.S. market through exports instead of via FDI. Since the

Table III.10   U.S. pharmaceutical trade through affiliates of foreign MNCs in the U.S.

PANEL A: U.S. imports through foreign MNCs affiliates in the U.S. (majority-owned)			
Imports current € millions	Total	% shipped directly from their own parents	of which European
1996	5,658	93.4	—
1997	5,986	91.9	—
1998	6,486	87.7	—
1999	7,209	90.9	—
2000	9,785	90.7	—
2001	10,725	—	—
2002	10,929	93.4	10,226
2003	12,028	91.1	11,625
2004	10,866	—	10,370

PANEL B: U.S. exports through foreign MNCs affiliates in the U.S. (majority-owned)			
Exports current € millions	Total	% shipped directly to their own parents	of which European
1996	3,324	85.8	—
1997	—	77.7	—
1998	3,679	70.2	—
1999	3,837	78.7	—
2000	5,961	76.2	—
2001	10,725	85.8	—
2002	6,114	77,7	5,854
2003	5,511	82.4	5,454
2004	5,418	—	5,343

Note: data for 2004 are preliminary

Source: BEA (2006)

Uruguay Round, this has occurred in the context of a general off-shoring trend, especially by the U.S. companies, followed by an increase of global outsourcing of the production of pharmaceutical active ingredients.

To a certain extent, U.S. FDI has fueled the positive growth performances of European countries such as Ireland, UK, Sweden, Hungary, and the Benelux. Figure III.4 reports the share of turnover of affiliates under foreign control in chemicals and pharmaceuticals (defined on the basis of the International Standard Industrial Classification—ISIC). Ireland, Hungary, Sweden, and UK have a turnover

Table III.11   U.S. net pharmaceutical imports through MNCs (majority-owned affiliates)

| | through affiliates sited | | Total |
	abroad of U.S. MNCs	in U.S. of foreign MNCs	
1996	-992 (-91)	2,334	1,342
1997	1,434 (-391)	—	—
1998	1,045	2,807	3,852
1999	1,690 (3,150)	3,372	5,062
2000	2,544 (4,223)	3,824	6,368
2001	4,474 (6,268)	—	—
2002	8,068 (9,178)	4,815 (4,372)	12,883 (13,550)
2003	1,055 (1,170)	6,517 (6,171)	7,490 (7,341)
2004	2,240 (2,028)	5,448 (5027)	7,688 (7,055)

Note: in parentheses, trade with Europe (U.S. MNCs sited in Europe and European MNCs in the U.S.).

Source: BEA (2006)

share higher than 80 percent.[14] In particular, foreign firms in Ireland accounted for 86 percent of net output in the manufacturing sector in 2000 and U.S.-controlled foreign enterprises contribute more than 90 percent of Irish chemical production.

Foreign firms can contribute to host economies through several channels. Table III.12 shows levels of U.S. outward stocks of pharmaceuticals and chemicals in Europe. It is clear that U.S. outward investments are mostly concentrated in those countries that have experienced the highest productivity growth rates, like the UK, Ireland and the Benelux (see Chapter II). These findings are in line with some econometric studies that have compared the productivity of foreign affiliates versus domestic firms controlling for size and sectoral effects. In fact, the main result is that foreign-owned subsidiaries are more productive if compared to local firms (Doms and Jensen, 1998; Criscuolo and Martin 2003; Barba Navaretti and Venables, 2004). In particular, Doms and Jensen (1998) using U.S. data, have settled on the following rank in terms of productivity levels: 1) U.S. MNCs; 2) non U.S. MNCs; 3) domestic non-MNCs. More recently, Criscuolo and Martin (2003) found the same ranking by analyzing UK data, showing that U.S. leadership seems to reflect a genuine competitive advantage of U.S. firms, independently from the actual firm's location.

---

[14] For Ireland and Hungary, the turnover share is available only in the chemical industry.

Figure III.4   Share of turnover of affiliates under foreign control in chemicals and pharmaceuticals (2001)

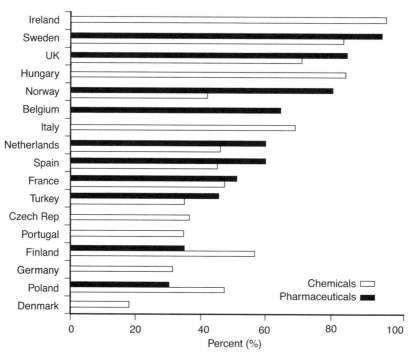

Note: Hungary and Italy and Denmark (1999); Czech Republic, Germany and Poland (2002), Belgium (2000, share of value added).

Source: our computations on OECD (2005), AmCham Belgium (2002).

More in general Helpman *et al.* (2004) find that "the least productive firms serve only the domestic market, that relatively more productive firms export, and that the most productive firms engage in FDI." This helps to explain, at least partially, poor productivity performances of the EU Mediterranean countries, which are characterized by higher market shares of domestic non-MNCs (see Table V.7).

Table III.13 compares different features of the pharmaceutical production and employment of U.S. affiliates abroad and of foreign affiliates in the U.S. Sales, value added, and number of employees of U.S. affiliates abroad greatly exceeds the correspondent values for foreign affiliates in the U.S. The opposite occurs for costs and labor productivity. What we observe could be due to a different type of FDI carried out by U.S. and EU firms. On the one hand, U.S. foreign direct

Table III.12 U.S. FDI outward stock in some European countries (€ millions)

Sectors		Belgium	France	Germany	Ireland	Italy	Nether.	Spain	Sweden	Switz.	UK
2004	P	2,601	3,571	841	—	1,599	1,274	1,126	—	2,045	5,740
	C	4,239	4,787	2,683	8,055	3,528	9,703	2,950	260	3,825	10,254
2003	P	2,691	2,804	985	—	1,527	1,277	962	—	1,704	5,943
	C	4,276	4,117	2,488	7,565	3,312	10,328	2,656	225	3,277	10,815
2002	P	3,106	1,162	881	—	1,216	—	822	—	1,496	6,670
	C	4,913	2,678	2,470	7,575	3,127	10,958	2,415	179	3,106	12,327
2001	P	2,530	1,536	—	—	1,009	2,023	358	—	1,648	4,830
	C	4,269	3,270	6,990	5,172	3,828	11,495	1,799	155	2,272	11,070
2000	P	3,011	2,458	475	—	806	2,317	366	—	—	5,644
	C	5,025	4,607	2,251	3,980	3,129	11,011	1,847	254	1,657	11,979
1995	P	—	1,519	1,204	—	852	312	202	—	—	1,737
	C	4,829	3,734	2,815	1,217	1,985	3,320	711	—	988	4,703
1990	P	923	818	517	—	671	138	177	—	—	568
	C	2,149	2,440	2,232	841	1,656	2,218	649	68	115	3,077

P = Pharmaceuticals, C = Chemicals

Source: BEA (2006)

investments in Europe are of the "vertical resource seeking" type, i.e. looking for the same productivity conditions of their home country (specifically, high capital/labor ratio and high labor productivity) but with lower labor costs per employee (see also Chapter II).

On the other hand, data from Table III.13 suggest that European investments in the U.S. are both horizontal "market seeking" and vertical "knowledge seeking" in R&D (where the U.S. has a competitive advantage). In fact, even though in absolute terms sales of U.S. MNCs in Europe are higher than those of European affiliates located in U.S., labor productivity of U.S. firms settled in Europe is far below the productivity of European firms located in the U.S. and U.S.-based companies in general. Evidence of R&D "resource seeking" is that affiliates of European firms in U.S. tend to invest more in R&D than U.S. MNCs in Europe.[15]

---

[15] According to BEA data, in 2003 European affiliates located in U.S. spent more than $7 million in R&D, while the total expenditure in R&D by U.S. multinationals abroad accounts for less than $5 million.

Table III.13   U.S. affiliates abroad versus foreign affiliates in the U.S. in pharmaceuticals: main indicators; 1998-2003[1]

		1998	1999	2000	2001	2002	2003
Number of employees	(A)	191	201.8	204.1	210.1	222.6	233.1
(thousands)	(B)	140.5	122.3	139.7	146.5	148.7	150
	(A)−(B)	50.2	79.5	64.4	63.6	73.9	83.1
Labor compensation	(A)	7,785	8,673	10,176	10,489	10,903	10,568
(€ millions)		9,909	9,550	13,115	14,841	14,998	16,516	—
	(A)−(B)	-2,124	-876	-2,939	-4,352	-4,095	-5,949
Sales	(A)	54,938	64,034	78,969	85,651	96,350	94,071
(€ millions)	(B)	46,151	47,361	63,563	70,338	73,237	66,775
	(A)−(B)	8,787	16,673	15,406	15,313	23,113	27,296
Value added	(A)	19,952	24,056	27,844	29,827	37,633	33,426
(€ millions)	(B)	15,948	14,369	20,246	21,086	23,045	24,908
	(A)−(B)	4,004	9,687	7,599	8,741	14,589	8,518
Labor cost per empl.	(A)	41	43	50	50	49	45
(€ thousands)	(B)	71	78	94	101	101	110
	(A)−(B)	-29	-35	-44	-51	-52	-65
Production per empl.	(A)	288	317	387	408	433	404
(€ thousands)	(B)	328	387	455	480	492	445
	(A)−(B)	-40	-70	-68	-73	-59	-42
value added per empl.	(A)	105	119	136	142	169	143
(€ thousands)	(B)	114	117	145	144	155	166
	(A)−(B)	-9	2	-9	-2	14	-23

(A)=U.S. affiliates abroad, (B)=foreign affiliates in the U.S.

(1)Only majority-owned affiliates considered.

Source:our computations on BEA (2006)

III.5   Size, Internationalization and Competitiveness

Large MNCs dominate the pharmaceutical industry. The huge sunk costs in R&D and clinical trials, along with considerable marketing expenditures, imply relevant economies of scale and scope. Related diversification and internationalization have always been the basic strategy in the sector to take full advantage of scale and scope economies both in terms of markets penetration and technology exploitation (Sutton 1998, Chandler 2005).

Table III.14 documents the on-going process of globalization within the industry: from 1998 to 2005 there is clear evidence of a decrease in market shares of local corporations in all major markets[16] (last column in Table III.14).

The headquarters of the most important pharmaceutical companies are located in the U.S., Western Europe and Japan. Nine of the top twenty companies, covering more than 60 percent of the worldwide market in 2005, are based in the U.S., six in EU-15, two in Switzerland, and in Japan.

EU-15 companies have lost almost 10 percent of the European market, while Japanese companies experienced a drop of more than 14 points in their domestic market shares. For the U.S., the reduction has been less pronounced, equal to 2.9 percentage points, indicating a higher ability of U.S. corporations to defend their domestic market shares. In fact, in 2005 the home market share of U.S. firms is around 10 percentage points higher than that of the EU-15 corporations (60.4 versus 50.8 percent). Within Europe, Germany is characterized by a high share of domestic corporations, totaling 36.1 percent of the German market. Japanese companies have retained about 64.1 percent of their domestic market, notwithstanding a sharp decline since 1998, when local market shares covered by national corporations were 78.4 percent. This high level of quotas in 1998 as compared to other countries seems to suggest a later opening of the Japanese market to foreign competitors.

By comparing the U.S. share in the EU-15 market to the EU-15 share in the U.S. market in 2005, we observe a higher penetration of U.S. corporations in Europe, the share being respectively 29 and 22.3 percent.

Looking at the most important European markets, the penetration of U.S. corporations is particularly high in the UK, Italy, and Spain, and lower in Germany and France.

U.S. multinationals have gained a significant fraction of the home market share lost by national companies (both European and Japanese companies) from 1998 to 2005, reflecting their increasing global penetration. The decline in the home market share of Japanese companies

---

[16] This result is in line with the increase of the trade openness ratio (see Table III.6).

Table III.14   Market shares in selected countries, by nationality of corporations (percent-%)

	1985	1989	1998	2002	2003	2004	2005	Δ'85-98	Δ'98-'05
U.S.									
U.S.	74.7	69.6	63.3	62.2	62.0	62.6	60.4	-11.4	-2.9
Japan	0.0	0.2	1.7	3.5	3.7	3.9	4.3	1.7	2.6
Switzerland	8.7	8.6	7.8	7.4	8.0	8.1	9.1	-0.9	1.3
EU-15	12.8	20.4	24.6	24.0	23.5	22.3	22.3	11.8	-2.3
Others	3.8	1.2	2.6	2.9	2.8	3.1	3.9	-1.2	1.3
Japan									
Japan	76.4	79.0	78.4	67.4	66.1	65.0	64.1	2.0	-14.3
U.S.	8.7	8.2	8.3	14.2	14.7	14.9	15.0	-0.4	6.7
Switzerland	3.3	3.6	3.6	7.2	7.7	8.0	8.4	0.3	4.8
EU-15	5.6	8.9	9.6	11.0	11.3	11.5	11.3	4.0	1.7
Others	6.0	0.3	0.1	0.3	0.3	0.5	1.2	-5.9	1.1
Germany									
Germany	56.6	55.0	45.1	40.8	41.1	38.2	36.1	-11.5	-9.0
Other EU-15	12.8	15.0	19.7	21.4	20.9	20.8	18.8	6.9	-0.9
U.S.	17.8	18.0	22.1	24.1	24.0	26.7	23.1	4.3	1.0
Japan	0.2	0.6	1.7	2.1	2.1	2.4	2.5	1.5	0.8
Switzerland	9.3	7.7	10.4	10.2	10.3	10.8	15.4	1.1	5.0
Others	3.3	3.7	1.1	1.5	1.7	1.2	4.1	-2.2	3.0
UK									
UK	33.4	42.7	24.5	22.8	20.3	18.9	19.0	-9.0	-5.5
Other EU-15	17.2	19.0	23.8	17.4	17.6	17.2	16.1	6.6	-7.7
U.S.	35.3	28.4	32.1	36.7	35.8	35.1	33.2	-3.2	1.1
Japan	0.0	0.0	0.9	2.0	2.1	2.3	2.5	0.9	1.6
Switzerland	7.0	6.5	7.3	7.5	7.6	7.7	7.5	0.3	0.2
Others	7.1	3.3	11.5	13.6	16.7	18.8	21.7	4.4	10.2
France									
France	51.6	48.5	36.9	32.8	32.0	30.6	30.2	-14.7	-6.7
Other EU-15	20.0	23.7	29.3	27.1	27.4	26.5	25.7	9.3	-3.6
U.S.	20.6	20.2	24.0	28.2	28.2	29.7	29.0	3.4	5.0
Japan	0.0	0.1	1.0	1.8	2.0	2.1	2.2	1.0	1.2
Switzerland	6.7	6.7	7.8	8.5	8.6	9.1	9.6	1.1	1.8
Others	1.1	0.9	1.1	1.6	1.8	2.0	3.3	0.0	2.2
Italy									
Italy	39.6	42.4	25.8	25.0	24.9	25.3	25.6	-13.8	-0.2
Other EU-15	27.8	27.3	32.4	31.2	30.9	29.9	31.1	4.6	-1.3
U.S.	17.6	19.3	27.1	30.0	29.9	29.4	28.3	9.5	1.2
Japan	0.0	0.2	1.2	1.7	1.7	1.8	1.8	1.2	0.6
Switzerland	9.4	9.1	12.6	10.7	11.1	11.3	10.6	3.2	-2.0
Others	5.6	1.6	1.0	1.5	1.5	2.3	2.6	-4.6	1.6

Table III.14   *continued*

	1985	1989	1998	2002	2003	2004	2005	Δ'85-98	Δ'98-'05
				Spain					
Spain	37.0	30.7	24.8	20.8	20.4	18.7	18.1	-12.2	-6.7
Other EU-15	32.6	38.1	40.0	36.3	36.0	34.9	33.9	7.4	-6.1
U.S.	15.3	16.8	23.6	31.3	31.5	33.3	33.1	8.3	9.5
Japan	0.1	0.1	1.3	1.4	1.5	1.5	1.6	1.2	0.3
Switzerland	12.2	11.6	9.4	8.9	9.3	10.1	10.5	-2.8	1.1
Others	2.8	2.7	1.0	1.2	1.4	1.6	2.8	-1.8	1.8
				EU-15[2]					
EU-15	—	—	60.5	55.0	54.6	52.8	50.8	—	-9.7
U.S.	—	—	26.1	29.9	29.7	30.4	29.0	—	2.9
Japan	—	—	1.2	1.7	1.8	1.9	2.0	—	0.8
Switzerland	—	—	9.6	9.3	9.6	9.9	11.1	—	1.5
Others	—	—	2.6	4.2	4.4	5.0	7.1	—	4.5

(1) Location of headquarters; data include hospital sales.

(2) The aggregate EU-15 has been calculated by weighting the market shares in respective countries by their market size. The aggregate does not include Luxembourg in 1998.

Source: IMS Health—World Review (various issues)

has not been counterbalanced by an increase of Japanese market shares in foreign markets as they have gained only 0.8 percentage points in Europe and 2.6 percentage points in the U.S.

The process of integration of the EU-15 market has cooled off with shares of EU-15 companies slightly decreasing in major European markets. This negative trend is particularly evident in the UK, where the share of other EU-15 companies dropped by 7.7 percent.

The Japanese market is an example of the differential performances of U.S. and EU-15 companies in the ability to penetrate international markets. EU-15 share in Japan has risen by 1.7 percent from 1998 to 2005, whereas U.S. corporations have gained 6.7 percentage points over the same period.

Table III.15 (above) and Table A.III.6 (in the Annex) show similar results for the top 100 companies.

In the period 1998-2005, U.S. corporations retained their national market shares and increased their penetration in Europe and other world markets. This result, together with the impressive growth of the

Table III.15   Global and regional market shares, by nationality of corporations (percent-%)

	1985	1989	1998	1999	2002	2003	2004	2005
U.S. Corporations								
World	34.2	31.2	36.0	39.0	41.5	40.7	40.2	38.4
North America	64.3	62.0	58.5	60.2	58.7	57.9	57.7	55.6
Europe	19.9	20.3	25.4	26.1	29.3	29.5	29.8	28.2
A/A/A (2)	11.4	11.1	12.3	14.4	16.3	16.5	16.6	16.1
Latin America	34.4	30.9	28.6	29.6	32.4	31.2	30.0	28.1
Japanese corporations								
World	13.1	15.7	11.0	11.1	8.1	7.9	7.7	7.7
North America	0.0	0.1	1.5	1.9	3.3	3.5	3.8	4.1
Europe	0.0	0.2	0.9	1.3	1.5	1.6	1.8	2.0
A/A/A	49.3	51.7	46.1	45.8	31.6	30.1	28.5	26.7
Latin America	0.0	0.0	0.2	0.2	0.4	0.4	0.4	0.5
EU-15 corporations								
World	24.8	24.7	28.8	27.8	26.7	27.1	26.0	27.1
North America	18.6	24.7	24.8	24.0	24.4	24.0	22.3	23.0
Europe	44.5	38.0	45.3	45.7	42.0	41.8	41.0	41.6
A/A/A	10.7	10.2	14.3	15.4	15.1	15.6	18.1	16.8
Latin America	22.9	22.8	27.8	26.7	26.6	26.5	26.7	27.4

Note: Based on Table A.III.6
Source: IMS Health—World Review (various issues)

U.S. market in the same period (see Table III.2), accounted for the good performance of U.S. corporations, which gained a 2.4 percent share of the world market for pharmaceuticals from 1998 to 2005 (5.5 percent to 2002; since then it has declined).

On the contrary, from 1998 to 2005, EU-15 corporations have lost ground in the European market (-3.7 percent), although they were able to contain their share reduction in the North American market (-1.8 percent), thus limiting a contraction of their world market share (-1.7 percent), which otherwise would have been more substantial.

The performance of EU-15 companies abroad changed significantly from 1985-1998 to 1998-2005. Indeed, while we observe an increase in market shares from 1985 to 1998, the reverse is true from 1998 to 2005. In 1985, the difference in world market shares between EU-15 and U.S. corporations was 9.4 percent; the gap increased to 11.3 percent in 2005.

Japanese companies are also losing ground at the global level, even if they have gained market share in Europe and in North America.

The wave of mergers and acquisitions at the end of the 1990s is reflected by the rapidly changing market shares of companies of European countries like France, Germany, UK and Sweden (see Table A.III.6). The acquisition of a Swedish company, Astra, by a British corporation, Zeneca, explains the rise of the market share recorded for the UK, and the corresponding decline of that of Sweden. Another example is Sanofi-Aventis (French), which is the cross-national consolidation of Hoechst (German), Sanofi-Synthelabo (French), Rhone-Poulenc (French), Rorer, Marion, Merrill and Dow (all U.S.) that occurred in two steps in 1998 and 2004. This operation could have affected the recent rise of the French market share and the decline of the German one.

The spurt of cross border mergers and acquisitions, together with the decline of home market share of local corporations, underscores the transnational consolidation of the pharmaceutical industry.

Economic integration has manifestly had an impact on aggregate trade flows, as we found by the gravity model in Section II. Here we perform a similar exercise at firm level. In particular, we evaluate the performances of MNCs in foreign markets,[17] controlling for the home market effect on total companies' sales. The dependent variable is given by the sales of each company "A" in any country "B" in U.S. dollars. Regressors include the total sales of multinational "A", i.e. the home market effect on foreign companies' performance, the total size of the market "B" as well as the distance[18] between the country where multinational "A" has placed its headquarter and the foreign national market "B" in which the MNC operates.

Table III.16 summarizes the results of a gravity regression model, where we analyze the sales in 28 national markets[19] by the top 200 pharmaceutical multinationals[20] in 2002.

---

[17] See box "Gravity Models".

[18] All values are expressed in natural logarithms. See box "Gravity Models" for details on distance calculation.

[19] The EU-25 (excluding Cyprus, Malta), U.S., Canada, China, India and Japan.

[20] We consider the top 200 companies by sales which are present in at least two national markets.

In the first version of the model the values of the coefficients of both the internal and the foreign market size are quite close to the theoretical values predicted by the gravity equation, whereas distance exerts the expected negative effect on MNC sales in foreign markets (see column 1 in Table III.16).

In the second regression (column 2) we add control variables for contiguous countries and for free trade areas (NAFTA and EU-15). Both dummies seem to have a negligible impact.

In Model 3 we add the number of ATC4 classes in which any given MNC is active, as a proxy of its level of diversification. Diversification has a positive and significant effect on internationalization. This is in line with what we expect as product diversification increases opportunities for the penetration of foreign markets.

Finally, in Model 4 we add nationality dummies for U.S. and EU-15 MNCs. Clearly, U.S. multinationals are outward oriented compared to European ones, while the opposite is true for EU-15 companies. Besides, by netting out the EU-15 nationality effect we detect a positive effect of the EU-15 market.

Summing up, there are two main findings.

First, even after controlling for the home market effect, U.S. multinationals perform better than their European competitors. The home market effect refers to an important result, proven both theoretically and empirically, in the international trade literature. According to that, a larger home market will attract disproportionately more firms, will produce a greater number of products, and therefore will enable home companies to become net exporters of differentiated goods. In this context, it means that U.S. MNCs penetrate foreign markets better than EU firms do, even after controlling for the large size of their domestic market.

Second, even if regional trade agreements have a positive effect on aggregate trade flows (see Table III.7), they do not seem to favor regional MNCs. In fact, according to the results in Table III.16, both NAFTA and EU do not affect firms' performance in foreign intra-regional markets. This result is particularly striking in the case of EU, given that its positive and significant impact on trade has been confirmed across different alternatives of the gravity model at the aggregate level.

Table III.16 Sales in foreign markets: gravity equation regression results

| Variable | Dep. var. Company's sales in foreign market (in logarithms) | | | |
	(1)	(2)	(3)	(4)
Company's sales[1]	1.0416‡	1.0432‡	1.0079‡	0.9777‡
	0.0250	*0.0250*	*0.0325*	*0.0337*
Market size[1]	0.9968‡	0.9887‡	0.9902‡	1.0030‡
	0.0249	*0.0269*	*0.0269*	*0.0273*
Distance[1]	-0.5773‡	-0.5427‡	-0.5284‡	-0.6599‡
	0.0423	*0.0579*	*0.0584*	*0.0707*
# of ATC4[1]	—	—	0.0013*	0.0017†
	—	—	*0.0007*	*0.0007*
U.S. companies	—	—	—	0.2730*
	—	—	—	*0.1509*
EU-15 companies	—	—	—	-0.2753*
	—	—	—	*0.1426*
Contiguous countries	—	-0.0171	-0.0288	-0.1462
	—	*0.1517*	*0.1518*	*0.1556*
NAFTA	—	-0.2150	-0.1707	-0.3912
	—	*0.3939*	*0.3946*	*0.4006*
EU-15	—	0.1572	0.1589	0.2557*
	—	*0.1217*	*0.1217*	*0.1308*
Constant	-16.1729‡	-16.3890‡	-16.1722‡	-14.8967‡
	0.4880	*0.5403*	*0.5548*	*0.6767*
N	2310	2310	2310	2310
R squared	0.5955	0.5959	0.5964	0.5983

(1) Logarithmic values

OLS regression. Marked coefficients are significant at: *10% level, † 5% level, ‡ 1% level.

Results have to be interpreted with caution, as regression results in Table III.16 are subject to a potential simultaneity problem since there is an accounting relationship between the dependent variable and both company and market size. This relationship tends to inflate the t values for these two regressors and R-squared, and to shadow correlations with other variables. To avoid potential misspecification problems, we transform the dependent variable and express the flow of sales from company "A" to country "B" as a deviation from a theoretical sales in case of no attrition.[21]

In formulas:

$$S_{AB} = \ln(F_{AB}) - \ln(F^*_{AB}) = \ln(F_{AB}) - (\ln(M_A) + \ln(M_B) - \ln(M_w))$$

where M_A is total sales of multinational "A", M_B is the total size of the market "B", M_w represents total world sales (used as a standardizing value) and F^* is the theoretical flow according to the gravity model assuming either perfect substitution between products of different firms on market "B" and no preference of firm "A" for any particular market absent trade frictions.

Table III.17 shows the results of the modified version of the gravity model. This model contains market dummies to take into account the potential impact of different market regulations in companies' decision to diversify geographically.[22] The estimated coefficient of distance has the expected sign: the smaller the distance between two countries the lower the deviation from the theoretical share.[23]

Controlling for total sales, size of the market, and geographical distance, U.S. companies are still able to penetrate into foreign markets better than EU-15 corporations (the results confirm the descriptive evidence reported in Table III.14, Table III.15, Table III.3, and Table A.III.6).

The inspection of the average residuals from the estimation of gravity model (3) in Table III.17 reveals that, in line with the empirical evidence previously discussed, U.S. multinationals are more competitive than EU companies. However, marked differences emerge across European countries. Danish, Dutch, Belgian and French companies are the most internationalized among the EU-15, with Dutch and Danish corporations displaying a higher market penetration than U.S. competitors. On the contrary, Spanish, Italian and German companies

---

[21] Another solution relies in the use of instruments for the regressors. We opt here for the simpler and use a transformation of the dependent variable. For clearer details on the gravity equation in case of zero trade costs see Helpman (1987) and Feenstra et al (1999).

[22] The number of observations in the regression raise from 2,310 (Table I.9) to 5,412 (Table I.10) since we take into account here also the values for which $F_{AB} = 0$, by letting $S_{AB} = -\ln(F^*_{AB})$.

[23] Since the theoretical share refers to the case of no friction, it is higher than the actual flow. Hence, $F_{AB} - F^*_{AB} \leq 0$. Therefore, according to the negative estimated coefficient, a decrease of distance reduces in absolute value the difference between the two flows.

Table III.17   Sales in foreign markets: "adjusted" gravity equation regression results

Variable	(1)	Dep. var.: Deviation from theoretical sales (2)	(3)	(4)
Distance	-1.2047‡	-1.2164‡	-1.1031‡	-1.4500‡
	0.0465	*0.0682*	*0.0667*	*0.0804*
Number of ATC4	—	—	0.0118‡	0.0119‡
	—	—	*0.0006*	*0.0007*
U.S. companies	—	—	—	1.8948‡
	—	—	—	*0.1310*
EU-15 companies	—	—	—	0.3522†
	—	—	—	*0.1568*
Contiguous Countries	—	0.2863	0.2414	0.0203
	—	*0.1951*	*0.1900*	*0.1899*
NAFTA	—	1.1239†	1.3710†	-0.3206
	—	*0.1951*	*0.5541*	*0.5683*
EU-15	—	-0.2596	-0.0023	-0.0645
	—	*0.1672*	*0.1635*	*0.1835*
Constant	—	3.6735‡	1.7695‡	4.7071‡
	—	*0.6717*	*0.6635*	*0.8275*
Dummies	>0† or >0‡	>0† or >0‡	>0† or >0‡	>0† or >0‡
	JPN <0†	JPN <0†	JPN <0†	JPN <0†
N	5412	5412	5412	5412
R squared	0.2298	0.2315	0.2713	0.2986

OLS regression. Coefficient marked are significant respectively at: *10% level, † 5% level, ‡ 1% level.

are inward oriented, i.e. they have not still been able to exploit the growing opportunities offered by foreign markets. This is not surprising if we interpret these results in light of their performance in terms of productivity. While Belgium, France and the Netherlands experienced a huge labor productivity growth in pharmaceuticals, higher than that of the U.S. (Table II.1), between 1996 and 2003, Spain, Italy and Germany lagged behind both in terms of productivity levels and growth rates. Thus, we find a positive relationship between internationalization and productivity in pharmaceuticals.

Among non-EU-15 countries, Japanese companies do not tend to expand into international markets. The new EU member states also display a common inward-oriented behavior.

In synthesis, the U.S. pharmaceutical industry is more competitive than the European one in terms of market size and production growth as well as internationalization through foreign direct investments and external market penetration.

The evidence produced in this chapter shows that the size of the U.S. market is not the only source of U.S. leadership, although it is an important factor. In fact, the benefits of domestic market size decrease with international integration (see Alesina and Spolaore, 2003). As the world pharmaceutical sector becomes more integrated, the benefits of large countries vanish in favor of smaller and more homogeneous countries. As for Europe, this fact can explain the positive growth performances of some of the small northern EU countries. However, if it is true that the globalization of the pharmaceutical industry reduces the advantages associated to the size of the market, the size of the market is an important factor driving the intensity of competitive and productivity growth. As a consequence, the administrative integration of the European market should be perceived as a priority for the future competitiveness of the European pharmaceutical industry.

Promoting the competitiveness of domestic industry must not be considered separately from the external challenge the new EU trade strategy will face in future years. From autumn 2006 and through 2007, the European Commission has set out the competitiveness agenda for EU trade policy with a series of linked initiatives. Among them, intellectual property rights (IPRs) enforcement will take a relevant role, especially towards a number of large countries like China (EU Commission, 2006).

Table A.III.1 is on the following pages.

Table A.III.2 Destination of pharmaceutical extra-EU exports (percent-%)

Exports of EU-15 from:	1986	1987	1988	1989	1990	1991	1992	1993	1994	1995	1996	1997	1998	1999	2000	2001	2002	2003	2004
EU-10[1]	4.7	4.1	4.2	3.9	2.8	4.2	4.7	5.7	6.9	7.4	8	8.2	8.4	7.7	7.5	7.7	7.4	7.7	8.2
U.S.	15.4	15.5	17.8	13.9	14.5	15.5	16.3	16	15.8	15.6	19.4	21	24.6	27.6	27.8	30.9	36.1	37.0	37.2
Switzerland	8.6	8.6	8.4	8.5	9.5	9.0	10.0	10.5	10.2	10.9	10.3	10.5	10.9	11.6	11.5	13.2	13.8	13.4	13.8
Japan	10.1	11.5	14.2	14.7	13.1	13.7	15	14.6	14.5	13.6	11.2	9.3	6.8	7.9	8.1	7.4	6.5	5.9	6.1
Canada	2.3	2.5	2.6	2.6	2.8	2.8	2.7	2.8	2.7	2.5	2.5	2.6	2.8	3.0	3.3	4.0	4.0	4.5	4.7
Rest of world	58.9	57.8	52.8	56.4	57.4	54.7	51.3	50.4	49.9	49.9	48.6	48.3	46.4	42.2	41.7	36.7	32.1	31.6	30.1

(1) New EU member states. Source: our computations on Table A.III.1.

Table A.III.3 Origin of pharmaceutical extra-EU imports (percent-%)

Imports of EU-15 from:	1986	1987	1988	1989	1990	1991	1992	1993	1994	1995	1996	1997	1998	1999	2000	2001	2002	2003	2004
EU-10	1.1	1.0	1.0	0.8	0.8	1.2	1.3	1.3	1.3	1.3	1.2	1.1	1.1	1.1	1.2	1.1	1.3	1.7	1.9
U.S.	34.8	31.2	31.5	32.7	31.3	32.3	31.9	33.5	33.5	34.5	39.6	42.8	46.6	48.4	52.4	56.5	55.6	56.0	55.9
Switzerland	46.2	48.2	48.8	47.6	49.1	48.3	47.2	45.1	44.7	42.7	39.5	36.2	35	32.5	27.4	23.8	24.8	23.6	24.6
Japan	6.4	6.4	6.5	6.6	6.4	6.6	7.6	7.7	7.4	7.9	7.4	7.1	5.6	5.7	5.7	5.2	4.5	4.8	4.4
Canada	0.6	0.6	0.6	0.8	1.2	1.2	1.1	1.6	2.0	1.5	1.2	1.1	1.0	1.1	1.0	0.8	1.0	2.0	1.7
Rest of world	10.9	12.5	11.6	11.5	11.1	10.4	10.9	10.9	11.1	12	11.2	11.7	10.8	11.1	12.2	12.6	12.8	11.9	11.5

(1) New EU member states. Source: our computations on Table A.III.1.

Table A.III.1　International trade in pharmaceutical products (€ millions)

	1986	1987	1988	1989	1990	1991	1992	1993	1994	1995	1996	1997	1998	1999	2000	2001	2002	2003	2004
PANEL A: EUROPE																			
EU-15 Exports																			
intra EU-15	6,448	6,834	7,895	9,209	10,240	12,150	13,785	14,513	17,128	19,736	21,017	24,392	28,225	32,918	38,993	47,849	72,142	74,410	81,978
extra EU-15	7,350	7,555	8,135	8,841	8,850	10,324	11,583	14,016	15,318	17,207	19,161	24,020	27,517	32,296	39,731	47,036	54,024	55,457	56,927
NAC	347	313	343	344	247	430	544	800	1,062	1,269	1,532	1,980	2,321	2,477	2,976	3,639	4,009	4,250	4,691
U.S.	1,133	1,168	1,445	1,232	1,280	1,604	1,894	2,247	2,425	2,692	3,715	5,043	6,771	8,907	11,045	14,541	19,528	20,528	21,152
Switzerland	635	650	684	748	838	932	1,163	1,477	1,562	1,884	1,972	2,526	2,987	3,758	4,583	6,232	7,457	7,427	7,841
Japan	740	871	1,157	1,303	1,163	1,418	1,733	2,043	2,214	2,337	2,146	2,243	1,880	2,567	3,224	3,467	3,500	3,263	3,468
Canada	165	188	210	232	244	292	311	385	408	437	479	635	779	966	1,331	1,886	2,163	2,475	2,668
Rest of world	4,329	4,363	4,295	4,982	5,079	5,647	5,938	7,063	7,648	8,589	9,318	11,593	12,779	13,621	16,572	17,271	17,367	17,514	17,109
Total	13,798	14,389	16,030	18,050	19,089	22,473	25,368	28,528	32,446	36,944	40,178	48,412	55,742	65,214	78,724	94,884	126,165	129,868	138,905
EU-15 Imports																			
intra EU-15	6,448	6,834	7,895	9,209	10,240	12,150	13,785	14,513	17,128	19,736	21,017	24,392	28,225	32,918	38,993	47,849	72,142	74,410	81,978
extra EU-15	2,980	3,092	3,426	4,010	4,436	5,120	5,881	6,812	7,386	8,452	9,689	11,076	12,878	14,995	17,928	22,860	24,963	25,312	29,974
NAC	32	32	31	31	37	60	78	85	97	112	117	123	139	169	216	255	332	434	561
U.S.	1,036	965	1,079	1,313	1,389	1,656	1,879	2,281	2,473	2,919	3,835	4,744	5,996	7,256	9,401	12,925	13,879	14,165	16,769
Switzerland	1,378	1,490	1,671	1,910	2,179	2,472	2,775	3,069	3,299	3,611	3,826	4,014	4,510	4,880	4,908	5,440	6,199	5,985	7,370
Japan	190	199	222	263	286	337	448	523	549	667	712	781	719	859	1,029	1,189	1,128	1,204	1,308
Canada	18	18	22	33	52	61	62	110	148	127	114	124	129	171	187	178	238	505	509
Rest of world	325	388	398	460	493	535	640	744	819	1,016	1,085	1,291	1,385	1,659	2,188	2,874	3,187	3,020	3,458
Total	9,428	9,926	11,321	13,219	14,676	17,270	19,666	21,325	24,515	28,189	30,706	35,468	41,103	47,913	56,920	70,709	97,105	99,723	111,953
Trade balance extra EU-15	4,370	4,463	4,709	4,831	4,414	5,203	5,702	7,203	7,932	8,755	9,472	12,944	14,640	17,302	21,804	24,176	29,061	30,145	26,953
Trade balance EU-15-U.S.	97	204	366	-81	-109	-52	15	-34	-48	-228	-120	299	775	1,651	1,645	1,617	5,649	6,363	4,383
PANEL B: U.S.																			
U.S. Exports																			
EU-25	1,049	976	1,090	1,319	1,394	1,668	1,905	2,326	2,530	2,995	3,936	4,890	6,155	7,453	9,652	13,266	14,246	14,553	17,048
EU-15	1,036	965	1,079	1,313	1,389	1,656	1,879	2,281	2,473	2,919	3,835	4,744	5,996	7,256	9,401	12,925	13,879	14,165	16,769
EU-10	14	11	11	6	5	13	26	45	56	75	101	146	159	197	252	341	367	387	279
Switzerland	48	55	50	60	58	86	122	244	410	243	217	484	454	803	919	1,199	1,028	890	1,094
Japan	623	580	654	719	610	672	658	830	792	849	821	895	885	1,045	1,175	1,357	1,366	1,208	1,214
Canada	279	260	267	316	339	430	564	744	771	745	880	1,152	1,360	1,750	2,387	2,445	2,514	2,529	2,421
Rest of world	720	671	697	733	756	937	1,083	1,211	1,287	1,314	1,706	2,075	2,412	2,893	3,369	4,064	3,770	3,596	3,592
Total	2,719	2,541	2,759	3,147	3,158	3,793	4,332	5,356	5,789	6,146	7,560	9,497	11,266	13,943	17,503	22,330	22,923	22,775	25,368

U.S. Imports

	1986	1987	1988	1989	1990	1991	1992	1993	1994	1995	1996	1997	1998	1999	2000	2001	2002	2003	2004
EU-25	1,159	1,188	1,456	1,239	1,289	1,613	1,905	2,258	2,437	2,706	3,731	5,066	6,806	8,934	11,082	14,586	19,614	20,750	21,317
EU-15	1,133	1,168	1,445	1,232	1,280	1,604	1,894	2,247	2,425	2,692	3,715	5,043	6,771	8,907	11,045	14,541	19,528	20,528	21,152
EU-10	26	19	11	7	10	9	11	10	12	15	16	23	34	27	37	45	87	222	166
Switzerland	187	229	304	295	327	366	473	474	512	553	581	774	844	981	1,140	1,515	1,436	1,377	1,167
Japan	249	276	270	197	170	220	254	342	385	402	499	640	803	1,235	1,665	1,806	1,985	2,130	1,814
Canada	53	51	58	65	79	95	133	168	261	281	338	576	585	660	903	1,271	1,308	1,647	1,713
Rest of world	383	312	300	123	126	199	208	330	387	340	479	720	756	995	1,288	1,761	1,961	2,153	2,424
Total	2,031	2,056	2,389	1,919	1,993	2,494	2,972	3,573	3,982	4,283	5,629	7,775	9,794	12,805	16,079	20,939	26,305	28,058	28,436
Trade Balance U.S.	688	485	370	1,228	1,165	1,300	1,360	1,783	1,807	1,863	1,931	1,722	1,473	1,138	1,424	1,391	-3,381	-5,283	-3,068

PANEL C: JAPAN

Japan Exports

	1986	1987	1988	1989	1990	1991	1992	1993	1994	1995	1996	1997	1998	1999	2000	2001	2002	2003	2004
EU-25	204	212	233	273	292	340	451	529	557	674	723	794	737	883	1,057	1,224	1,169	1,243	1,333
EU-15	190	199	222	263	286	337	448	523	549	667	712	781	719	859	1,029	1,189	1,128	1,204	1,308
EU-10	13	13	11	11	7	3	3	6	8	8	11	13	18	24	28	36	41	39	26
Switzerland	10	8	8	9	6	9	7	21	14	16	23	32	35	45	62	103	110	102	126
U.S.	249	276	270	197	170	220	254	342	385	402	499	640	803	1,235	1,665	1,806	1,985	2,130	1,814
Canada	8	7	8	9	6	6	8	16	24	25	31	31	29	30	19	15	27	26	44
Rest of world	205	241	281	307	318	396	412	477	474	497	517	577	530	630	735	717	684	641	632
Total	675	745	800	795	794	971	1,132	1,385	1,455	1,614	1,793	2,074	2,134	2,823	3,538	3,866	3,976	4,142	3,950

Japan Imports

	1986	1987	1988	1989	1990	1991	1992	1993	1994	1995	1996	1997	1998	1999	2000	2001	2002	2003	2004
EU-25	760	887	1,177	1,325	1,178	1,435	1,749	2,058	2,232	2,346	2,159	2,257	1,886	2,575	3,232	3,475	3,507	3,270	3,474
EU-15	740	871	1,157	1,303	1,163	1,418	1,733	2,043	2,214	2,337	2,146	2,243	1,880	2,567	3,224	3,467	3,500	3,263	3,468
EU-10	20	15	19	23	16	17	15	15	17	10	13	13	6	8	8	7	7	7	6
Switzerland	240	240	280	285	312	267	254	264	270	293	308	297	295	350	334	347	366	557	584
U.S.	623	580	654	719	610	672	658	830	792	849	821	895	885	1,045	1,175	1,357	1,366	1,208	1,214
Canada	4	7	7	7	5	5	19	23	40	43	40	40	34	40	50	53	55	33	35
Rest of world	124	114	129	142	121	133	149	179	214	226	216	251	245	298	377	409	444	406	413
Total	1,750	1,827	2,247	2,478	2,226	2,512	2,828	3,355	3,548	3,758	3,544	3,740	3,344	4,309	5,168	5,640	5,738	5,475	5,719
Trade Balance Japan	-1,075	-1,082	-1,447	-1,683	-1,432	-1,541	-1,696	-1,970	-2,093	-2,143	-1,751	-1,667	-1,210	-1,486	-1,630	-1,774	-1,762	-1,333	-1,769

Our elaborations on the NBER-UN World Trade database (1986-2000) and UN Comtrade (2001-2004) database. For consistency data for exports are based on imports of partner countries.

Table A.III.4   U.S. exports of chemicals to MNC affiliates in Europe (majority-owned)

	1996	1997	1998	1999	2000	2001	2002	2003
Europe	4,084	5,140	4,598	5,695	7,191	6,399	5,552	7,432
Austria	2	5	3	1	1	1	—	—
Belgium	979	1,137	926	835	849	553	489	595
Czech Republic	—	—	—	1	1	4	2	2
Denmark	—	4	4	8	—	—	23	15
Finland	—	13		14	19	16	15	11
France	564	510	590	1,030	1,462	1,303	871	956
	160	*142*	*—*	*290*	*—*	*—*	*—*	*—*
Germany	417	414	340	479	601	583	585	425
	98	*150*	*83*	*29*	*43*	*99*	*65*	*76*
Greece	5	2	—	—	—	—	—	2
Hungary	—	—	—	4	10	6	6	4
Ireland	131	248	468	483	475	402	504	365
Italy	243	295	231	235	355	392	256	591
Luxembourg								
Netherlands	535	99	555	724	1,456	1,504	1,207	1,058
	—	*—*	*9*	*—*	*—*	*17*	*—*	*—*
Norway	—	—	—	5	—	18	—	—
Poland	—	—	—	5	4	3	2	2
Portugal	6		2	—	1	—	—	1
Russia	—	—	—	—	1	3	3	3
Spain	139	150	211	90	170	144	168	126
Sweden	57	—	32	49	—	90	86	—
Switzerland	102	103	78	73	77	76	82	—
Turkey	1	—	1	1	13	13	3	4
United Kingdom	883	1,205	1,114	1,634	1,598	1,257	1,226	1,325
	217	*379*	*497*	*473*	*339*	*408*	*647*	*868*
Other	6	—	—	2	—	3	—	4

Note: Pharmaceutical exports in *italics*

Source: BEA (2006)

Table A.III.5   U.S. imports of chemicals to MNC affiliates from Europe (majority-owned)

	1996	1997	1998	1999	2000	2001	2002	2003
Europe	2,437	2,901	5,009	6,792	8,697	11,080	14,810	7,860
Austria	—	3	2	—	—	—	—	—
Belgium	448	482	425	631	444	450	440	376
Czech Republic	—	—	—	—	—	—	4	5
Denmark	—	6	7	—	35	36	63	47
Finland	—	—	—	—	—	—	92	
France	217	283	258	369	620	681	625	651
	23	*19*	*26*	*138*	—	—	—	—
Germany	248	340	216	292	389	413	511	400
	18	*44*	*13*	*19*	*14*	—	*104*	*65*
Greece	1	1	1	—	—	—	—	—
Hungary	—	—	—	1	1	1	1	1
Ireland	488	520	2,805	3,594	4,858	6,987	10,502	4,059
Italy	180	21	78	123	219	290	361	241
Luxembourg	—	—	—	—	—	—	—	—
Netherlands	169	276	269	357	665	700	641	499
	2	*24*	—	*57*	*214*	*55*	*60*	*88*
Norway	—	—	—	—	41	37	—	—
Poland	—	—	1	—	2	—	—	—
Portugal	2	1	38	1	2	1	—	—
Russia								
Spain	27	47	—	91	119	138	99	68
Sweden	—	—	172	—	—	—	—	—
Switzerland	44	183	—	82	109	95	97	55
Turkey	—	—	—	—	1	—	—	—
United Kingdom	521	430	420	943	995	861	1,093	962
	139	*147*	*157*	*525*	*340*	*270*	*641*	*583*
Other	1	—	—	—	15	—	—	—

Note: Pharmaceutical exports in *italics*

Source: BEA (2006)

Table A.III.6   Shares of top 100 corporate groups, by nationality of corporation and major markets (%), 1985-2005

Markets	U.S.	JAP	SWI	EU-15	GER	UK	FRA	ITA	SWE	DEN	NET	BEL
				Nationality of corporation [1]								
1985												
World	34.2	13.1	7.7	24.8	9.6	9.2	2.8	1.3	0.6	0.2	0.5	0.6
North America	64.3	0.0	8.8	18.6	4.3	12.9	0.2	0.6	0.1	0.0	0.2	0.3
Europe	19.9	0.0	8.5	44.5	18.1	10.6	7.9	3.5	1.5	0.5	1.1	1.3
A/A/A [2]	11.4	49.3	4.8	10.7	5.8	3.7	0.5	0.1	0.1	0.0	0.3	0.2
Latin America	34.4	0.0	11.1	22.9	14.8	4.5	2.2	0.5	0.1	0.0	0.6	0.2
1989												
World	31.2	15.7	10.1	24.7	9.6	7.4	3.2	2.1	1.0	0.4	0.5	0.5
North America	62.0	0.1	5.2	24.7	14.0	8.8	0.2	0.5	0.5	0.2	0.2	0.3
Europe	20.3	0.2	17.3	38.0	11.3	8.3	8.1	5.2	2.4	0.7	1.0	1.0
A/A/A	11.1	51.7	6.6	10.2	4.0	4.4	0.7	0.2	0.4	0.1	0.3	0.1
Latin America	30.9	0.0	15.9	22.8	5.7	12.0	3.3	1.0	0.2	0.0	0.6	0.0
1998												
World	36.0	11.0	8.0	28.8	10.0	9.0	4.4	0.6	2.8	0.7	0.6	0.6
North America	58.5	1.5	7.9	24.8	6.8	11.6	1.8	0.0	3.5	0.2	0.4	0.5
Europe	25.4	0.9	9.6	45.3	15.3	10.2	9.8	1.8	3.7	1.7	0.9	1.5
A/A/A	12.3	46.1	5.1	14.3	6.3	4.1	1.7	0.0	0.9	0.8	0.3	0.2
Latin America	28.6	0.2	11.9	27.8	16.1	5.8	4.1	0.1	0.7	0.0	1.0	0.0
1999												
World	39.0	11.1	7.7	27.8	7.3	11.9	6.1	0.5	0.0	0.7	0.6	0.6
North America	60.2	1.9	7.6	24.0	4.8	14.9	3.0	0.0	0.0	0.3	0.5	0.5
Europe	26.1	1.3	9.5	45.7	12.3	13.8	13.0	2.1	0.0	1.7	0.9	1.5
A/A/A	14.4	45.8	5.1	15.4	4.6	5.5	3.8	0.0	0.0	0.9	0.4	0.2
Latin America	29.6	0.2	11.7	26.7	12.1	6.6	6.7	0.2	0.0	0.1	0.9	0.1
2002												
World	41.5	8.1	8.0	26.7	6.1	12.0	5.7	0.5	0.0	0.9	0.6	0.6
North America	58.7	3.3	7.5	24.4	3.7	15.0	3.8	0.1	0.0	0.4	0.5	0.5
Europe	29.3	1.5	9.4	42.0	11.6	12.2	11.5	1.9	0.0	2.2	0.8	1.2
A/A/A	16.3	31.6	7.1	15.1	4.2	5.7	3.6	0.1	0.0	0.8	0.4	0.3
Latin America	32.4	0.4	11.8	26.6	11.4	6.7	6.8	0.1	0.0	0.2	1.0	0.3
2003												
World	40.7	7.9	8.4	27.1	6.6	11.3	6.2	0.7	0.0	1.0	0.6	0.6
North America	57.9	3.5	7.9	24.0	4.3	14.0	4.1	0.2	0.0	0.5	0.4	0.5
Europe	29.5	1.6	9.7	41.8	12.0	11.3	11.6	2.2	0.0	2.0	1.1	1.1
A/A/A	16.5	30.1	7.3	15.6	4.2	5.9	3.9	0.1	0.0	0.8	0.4	0.3
Latin America	31.2	0.4	11.9	26.5	11.3	6.5	6.7	0.2	0.0	0.3	1.1	0.3
2004												
World	40.2	7.7	8.6	26.0	6.2	10.6	6.1	0.7	0.0	1.1	0.5	0.7
North America	57.7	3.8	8.1	22.3	3.8	12.9	4.1	0.1	0.0	0.5	0.2	0.7
Europe	29.8	1.8	10.0	41.0	11.9	11.0	11.0	2.2	0.0	2.1	1.1	1.2
A/A/A	16.6	28.5	7.6	18.1	6.3	6.1	3.9	0.1	0.0	0.9	0.5	0.3
Latin America	30.0	0.4	11.4	26.7	11.5	6.4	6.6	0.2	0.0	0.5	1.0	0.4
2005												
World	38.4	7.7	9.3	27.1	6.4	10.8	6.3	0.8	0.0	1.3	0.5	0.9
North America	55.6	4.1	9.1	23.0	3.7	13.3	4.2	0.1	0.0	0.7	0.2	0.8
Europe	28.2	2.0	11.1	41.6	12.0	10.7	11.1	2.6	0.0	2.4	1	1.3
A/A/A	16.1	26.7	7.8	16.8	4.4	6.3	4.1	0.2	0.0	0.9	0.5	0.4
Latin America	28.1	0.5	10.2	27.4	12.4	6.1	6.5	0.3	0.0	0.5	1	0.5

1. Location of headquarters. 2. Africa, Asia and Australasia.

Source: IMS Health—World Review (various issues)

Appendix III.2

Tax Incentives and Foreign Direct Investments: The Irish Case

One of the most important factors influencing economic growth is investment in capital goods (Jorgenson and Yun, 2001). Further, the adoption of new technologies strongly depends on the willingness to purchase new equipments and assets. Among the many factors that influence investment decisions, the tax burden has a significant negative impact. Recently, an analysis based on many empirical studies has shown that cross-border investment is highly sensitive to tax rates: an increase of one percentage point in the corporate income-tax rate causes the stock of foreign direct investment to decline by more than three percent (de Mooij and Ederveen 2003).

Business investment decisions are affected among others by taxes on corporate income, capital taxes, labor taxes, sales taxes on business inputs and other capital-related taxes. The marginal effective tax rate is a summary measure of the extent to which taxes impinge on investment decisions. It is the share of the pre-tax return on capital that would be required to cover the taxes, leaving a residual to cover the costs of debt and equity used to finance capital investments (Mintz *et. al.*, 2005). According to the marginal effective tax rate on capital for large and medium-size corporations, Ireland ranks at the bottom of the list of OECD countries and leading developing countries.

The introduction in Ireland in the late 1950s of a zero tax rate on profits derived from exports in the manufacturing sector, led firms from continental Europe and especially the U.S. to adopt Ireland as an export platform. Ireland's low corporate tax rate of 12.5 percent on trading profits has been a magnet for MNCs who are responsible for 90 percent of Irish exports. Before the tax change, Ireland had an export comparative advantage only in the food, beverages and tobacco sectors. Upon accession to the EU in 1992, Ireland was the EU member with the lowest corporate tax rate and had gained an export comparative advantage in chemicals, and particularly in pharmaceuticals, thus becoming well established as a European production base and export platform for foreign multinationals (see Lipsey 2003).[24] A low tax environment attracts real foreign direct investment but might also

---

[24] There were equivalent FDI booms in Spain and Portugal following their accession in the 1980s but, by the mid-1990s, the share of FDI in these economies began to stabilize at much lower levels than in the Irish case.

increases nominal investments by providing incentive to shift profits to the low tax location via transfer pricing (Honohan and Walsh, 2002; Blanchard, 2002). While clearly influencing total FDI inflows, a low rate of corporation tax also influences the types of sectors an economy attracts. Transfer pricing arises where arm's-length trading prices are difficult to establish. This is particularly the case for R&D and advertising intensive sectors, since these factors make it difficult to locate the exact source of value added.[25] Apart from tax advantages, Ireland has proved to be a particularly attractive location for U.S. corporations for a number of factors: its status of an English-speaking country, its geographic location and the cultural connections with the Irish-American business community. By the late 1990s, nine of the top ten pharmaceutical companies in the world had operations in Ireland. Pfizer was one of the first U.S. pharmaceutical businesses to locate in Ireland and set up its first production facility in Ringaskiddy in 1969 to produce food chemicals. The dominant influence behind the company's decision to locate in Ireland at the time was an Irish emigrant who held one-third of the company's shares. Since then, Pfizer has opened nine operating plans in Ireland and today it employs around 2,200 people in Dublin and Cork. Ireland has been growing in importance not just as a base from which U.S. companies export to the EU but also as a base from which they export back to the U.S.

Ireland is the most profitable location of U.S. multinationals and in the period 1998-2002, the profits of U.S. companies with Irish facilities doubled from $13.4 to 26.8 billion, while profits in most of the rest of Europe dropped.[26] Altshuler *et. al.* (2001) estimates of the tax elasticity of U.S. FDI flows suggest that the stock of U.S. manufactur-

---

[25] Moreover, Ireland's tax exemption in respect of certain patent royalties, has been one of the driving factors behind investment by pharmaceutical multinationals, principally from the U.S., in the Irish economy. Irish tax legislation provides an exemption from tax for income derived from "qualifying patents" when received by a person resident in Ireland and not resident in any other country. Patent royalties received by patent holders will be exempt from Irish corporation tax, and dividends paid on the ordinary shares of the patent holding company, or on other shares but only to the inventor or co-inventor, will be exempt from Irish income tax in the hands of the shareholders.

[26] Profits booked abroad—mostly in low-tax jurisdictions—do not fully reflect shifts in where companies do business. In particular, in October 2004, the Financial Times emphasized that from 1994 to 2003, foreign profits of the six largest U.S. pharmaceuticals companies went from 38 percent of their overall income to more than 65 percent. At the same time, the taxes paid on those profits fell from a rate of 31 percent to 17.5 percent, just half the U.S. corporate tax rate. Even as their overseas share of profits nearly doubled over the past decade, their overseas sales grew from just 40 to 43 percent.

ing investment in Ireland is 70 percent higher than it would have been if Ireland had a tax rate equal to the next lowest EU rate. The effect is even more dramatic, of course, if compared with the average EU tax rate. Gropp and Kostinal (2000) come to a similar conclusion that about 80 percent of Ireland's net FDI inflow would disappear if rates were harmonized at the average EU level.

Chapter IV
R&D and Innovation

Chapter IV
R&D and Innovation

Main Findings

- Beginning in the mid-1990s, R&D productivity has experienced a downturn worldwide. Because of the geographical concentration of R&D activities in the U.S., this productivity decline partially explains the slowdown in U.S. productivity performances in pharmaceuticals (see Chapter II).

- Despite increasing private and public pharmaceutical R&D, the number of new active substances launched into the market was substantially stable in the first half of the 1990s and turned downward afterwards.

- During the 1990s, attrition rates of R&D projects in pharmaceuticals increased, especially in clinical phases II and III.

- Besides stringent requirements for clinical trials imposed by the regulatory authorities in the U.S. and Europe, the increase of attrition rates of drug candidates can be attributed to a high degree of complexity of R&D activities (intensely targeted toward complex pathologies such as diseases with multifactorial or unknown etiology, chronic or lethal diseases). It implies an increase in the resources and capabilities needed for successful drug development.

- Relevant scientific knowledge and organizational skills in pharmaceuticals have broadly dispersed since the molecular biology revolution in the second half of the 1970s. No single organization has been able to internally master and control all the competencies required to develop new drugs. As a result, the division of innovative labor has grown exponentially (see, Arora and Gambardella, 1994b, Orsenigo *et al.*, 2001). The number of inventors, assignees and backward citations per patent, as well as the number of licensing agreements and other collaborative agreements has soared.

- We argue that R&D productivity slowdown might be explained by multiple concurrent factors:

1. R&D exhaustion (the "fishing out" effect);

2. Genomics and general purpose technologies;

3. Gestation lags and time to market;

4. Poor market incentives for innovation (see Chapter IV).

Moreover, there might be measurement drawbacks related to the fact that all available measures of R&D input and output are only imperfect proxies for innovation.

- In a scenario of decreasing returns to R&D investments, the U.S. research system ranks first in terms of total public and private R&D, as well as public and private R&D intensity. The data clearly show the U.S. corporate superior innovative performance: U.S. firms hold the majority of biopharmaceutical patents (with an increasing importance over time), are more specialized in the biotechnology domain and play a pivotal role in the international network of division of innovative labor. In addition, U.S. corporations are leaders in terms of the number and sales of New Molecular Entities (NMEs), whereas European companies are experiencing a competitive disadvantage in selling their new drugs.

- China and India are consolidating their scientific and technological capabilities in the life sciences and in pharmaceuticals, as documented by trends of scientific publications and patents, posing a warning for European industry.

- Biopharmaceutical R&D is increasingly globalized, with the U.S. research system occupying a prominent position in the international network of division of innovative labor.

- The U.S. innovation system is by far the most advanced: public research organizations and small biotechnology companies play a critical role in integrating explorations of new research trajectories with clinical needs, sustaining the expansion of R&D activities on neglected, niche, and new pharmaceutical markets.

- The growth of the U.S. biotechnology sector was supported by the evolution of the U.S. capital markets and institutions.

The stock market and venture capital investment boom of the late 1990s greatly increased the favorable conditions for the flourishing of new biotech start-ups and the internationalization of the venture capital industry which was hitherto a U.S. phenomenon. However, whereas in Europe the bubble burst caused a significant blow to biotech share prices, in the U.S. the situation was quite different. There, the fine-grained R&D network and the highly competitive price structure constituted the breeding ground for the real beginning of a new industrial sector, capable of continuing its activities well after the bursting of the high tech bubble. U.S. institutions play a crucial role: transparent and deep markets and networks for human resources, capital and knowledge explain the structural advantage of the U.S. industry as compared to the cyclical performances of the EU innovation system.

IV.1 Overview

In this chapter, we present the global trends in R&D productivity of the pharmaceutical industry over the last 30 years, combining data from various sources to evaluate firm innovative performances.

Technological change is an important source of long-run productivity growth and competitiveness in pharmaceuticals, with deep implications as far as welfare and living standards are concerned. Even if the empirical studies on the returns to R&D present mixed evidence (Griliches, 1998), most of them find a robust relationship between total factor productivity and such measures as R&D outlays, percentage of sales from innovative products and number of patents (Griliches, 1980, 1984; Griliches and Mairesse, 1983; Lichtenberg and Siegel, 1991; Hall and Mairesse, 1995; Crepon, *et al.* 1998; Lööf and Heshmati, 2001). However, despite public and private R&D expenditures in pharmaceuticals growing exponentially during the last thirty years, the rate at which the industry has generated New Molecular Entities (NMEs) is not growing. It has been substantially stable over the 1990s, with a steep decrease since 1996.

The causes of this phenomenon are under debate. Some studies point to the propensity of some pharmaceutical companies to control for risk by pursuing less innovative research, while others blame stricter regulation policies. This is especially the case of FDA, as the introduction of increasing stringent requirements for clinical trials implies larger, more costly and internationally based clinical trials and an increase in the resources, both in terms of R&D effort and capabilities, needed to develop new drugs.

In the next section we discuss the reasons why research inputs have grown so rapidly whereas new drug launches have not, arguing that the slowdown of R&D productivity in pharmaceuticals is related to the growing complexity (and costs) of the R&D process and goals. On the one side, R&D projects are more and more focused on complex pathologies. On the other side, the organizational shifts that characterized the industry since the advent of biotechnology have forced companies to rely on a wide network of collaborations in order to access the different resources and capabilities needed in the drug innovation process, but that are widely dispersed across a variety of different actors (see Arora and Gambardella, 1994b, Orsenigo *et al.* 2001).

The Slowdown of R&D Productivity in Pharmaceuticals

1. R&D effort has increased, while the number of new molecular entities has declined

Figure IV.1 reports the trends of public and private R&D expenditure carried out in the U.S. during the last thirty years.

A steep increase characterizes both public and private expenditure: since the beginning of the 1990s private-sector pharmaceutical R&D spending tripled and public sector support doubled.[1]

Despite the exponential growth of public and private R&D expenditures in pharmaceuticals over the last 30 years, the rate at which the industry has generated NMEs appears to be substantially stable over the 1990s and shows a decreasing trend in the latest years (see Figure IV.1).

NMEs are novel substances with pharmacological activity launched on the world market for the first time and represent the preferred

---

[1] U.S. trends are highlighted; further analysis in the following section, however, shows that the increase in R&D spending is a global trend.

Figure IV.1   U.S. Pharmaceutical R&D spending (right axis) and New Molecular Entities approved by the FDA (left axis), 1976-2004

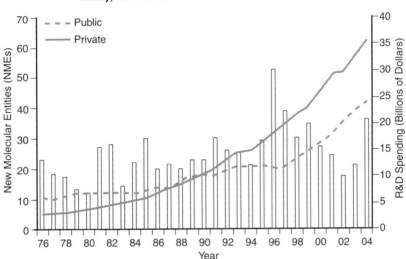

Note: Lines denote U.S. private and public R&D spending in inflation-adjusted to constant 2002 U.S. dollars by the National Institutes of Health (NIH) Biomedical R&D price deflator.

Source:U.S. Food and Drug Administration, Center for Drug Evaluation and Research. The 2004 figure includes new therapeutic biologic products transferred from CBER to CDER. For R&D spending, OECD, ANBERD Database and U.S. budget.

indicator of research outcome from innovative activities in the pharmaceutical sector. On the one side, R&D effort, as measured by R&D expenditures, has increased, whereas the number of NMEs launched has remained stable or decreased over time, leading to a decrease in the productivity of R&D activities.

2. Attrition rates of R&D projects have risen

In order to measure attrition rates, we identify two possible outcomes for R&D projects: success and failure. Success is defined as a transition from one phase of drug development to the next one, while a project is considered to be failed if it has been discontinued, suspended or it is stated to be no longer in active research.

Figure IV.2 reports the share of successful projects over the total number of projects entering in any given phase of R&D in a certain

Figure IV.2   The probability of success of pharmaceutical R&D projects by stage of development, 1990-2000

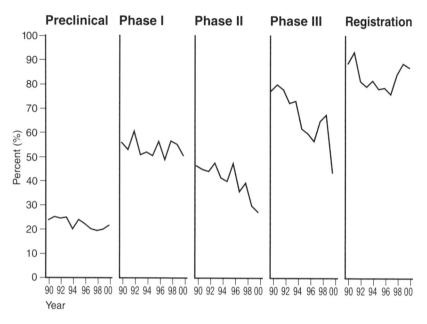

Source: our computations on Databiotech.com

year, where the horizontal axis represents the year of entry into the stage considered in each subplot.

Estimation of attrition rates is complicated by the fact that the process of drug development is extremely lengthy. Based on a survey of ten large pharmaceutical companies, DiMasi *et al.* (2003) estimated the mean time from phase I to submission of a New Drug Application with the FDA to be about six years (12.3 months for completing Phase I, 26.0 months for Phase II, and 33.8 months for Phase III). Using a more comprehensive dataset, Abrantes *et al.* (2003) states that for drugs that successfully passes through all three phases of clinical development, the whole process takes on average (not including any time spent between phases) 8 years. The time required for the assessment involved in each stage does not allow us to produce a sound estimation of the probability of success for projects that started a given phase after the year 2000. Therefore, we assume that projects that entered preclinical or clinical trials before 2000 and have not yet moved on are failed.

Figure IV.2 shows that during the 1990s, the attrition rate of pharmaceutical R&D projects increased, especially in clinical phases II and III (see also Mervis, 2005). In clinical phase II, the probability of success has dropped from almost one half to less than one third while projects that started phase III in year 2000 have a probability of success that is almost one half than that of projects that entered phase III ten years before.

3. R&D efforts are more intensely directed towards complex pathologies

To understand the direction of R&D endeavors in the last decade, we analyzed the distribution of private R&D activities within specific therapeutic areas. We considered the distribution of new therapeutic activities by public research organizations (PROs), established pharmaceutical companies (ECs) and dedicated biotechnology firms (DBFs), i.e. therapeutic indications in which the firm or institution was not active before 1995.

Databiotech.com provides information about R&D projects reporting the name of the company that originated the compound, the name of the licensee(s), if any, and a description of the therapeutic indication(s) targeted by the compound under development. Moreover, detailed information about the time of entry into each stage involved in clinical development is reported.

Data have been organized in a matrix. Rows represent the firms and public institutions, whereas columns correspond to indications. Each cell corresponds to the number of active projects started by the row-institution targeting the column-indication. We construct two different matrices: the 1995-matrix only considers the projects started up to the year 1995, whereas the 2005-matrix considers the project started from 1995 to 2005. The comparison of the 1995-matrix with the 2005-matrix provides information about change in the allocation of R&D efforts[2].

Table IV.1 reports the intensity of entry into therapeutic indications classified according to their characteristics in terms of etiology, diffu-

---

[2] Sembenelli and Vannoni (2000) apply a similar approach to the study of the firms' entry strategies into different industries.

Table IV.1   Change in complexity of R&D efforts in terms of the characteristics of targeted disease states

Disease Characteristics		Potential Entry	Actual Entry	Intensity %				Avg Success Rate %
				Tot.	PRO	DBF	EC	
Etiology	Monofactorial	289,628	1,755	0.61	0.51	0.79	0.72	21.67
	Unknown	50,656	451	0.89	0.50	1.25	1.56	20.35
	Multifactorial	565,866	7,279	1.29	0.92	1.73	1.61	17.22
Chronicity	Acute	299,429	1,839	0.61	0.41	0.85	0.89	19.89
	Chronic	604,175	7,624	1.26	0.95	1.68	1.53	17.58
Outcome	Not lethal	256,138	1,630	0.64	0.38	0.84	1.09	21.00
	Maybe lethal	485,837	5,118	1.05	0.78	1.44	1.28	17.62
	Always lethal	164,175	2,737	1.67	1.33	2.15	1.78	16.51
Diffusion	Rare	213,642	1,206	0.56	0.38	0.78	0.80	36.20
	Widespread	689,956	8,269	1.20	0.89	1.60	1.49	16.96

PRO=Public Research Organization; DBF=Dedicated Biotech Firm; EC=Established companies, mostly pharmaceutical companies.

Source: our computations on Databiotech.com

sion, and outcome, as a proxy for their difficulty.[3] "Potential Entry" is equal to the hypothetical number of projects that would have been started in the case that all the firms would have entered all the areas in which they were not active before 1995. "Actual Entry" is the number of new therapeutic areas in which pharmaceutical companies entered since 1995. The intensity of entry into the therapeutic categories is computed by taking the ratio of actual entry over potential entry. The intensity of entry is further classified on the basis of the typology of firm, distinguishing PROs, DBFs, and ECs.

Table IV.1 reports also the rate of success of the R&D projects according to the characteristics, in terms of outcome, etiology, and diffusion, of the therapeutic indication.

By comparing the rate of activity and the probability of success, we find out that R&D projects are more intensely target toward complex pathologies (i.e. pathologies with a lower average probability of successful development):

---

[3] According to our definition, a firm starts a new therapeutic activity when it enters a therapeutic indication in which it was not active before 1995.

- diseases with multifactorial or unknown etiology;

- chronic diseases;

- diseases that are always lethal or that can be lethal if not treated;

- largely diffused diseases.[4]

The result does not change substantially by typology of organization, even though the analysis highlights a higher involvement of biotechnology companies into projects targeting pathologies more complex, in particular lethal and chronic diseases.

4. The division of innovative labor has increased

The explosion of knowledge in molecular biology and genetics has generated a wide range of new therapeutic opportunities. Because the relevant scientific knowledge and organizational skills are broadly dispersed, no single organization has been able to internally master and control all the competencies required to develop a new medicine (Powell *et al.* 1996, Pammolli *et al.* 2000, Orsenigo *et al.* 2001, Owen-Smith *et al.* 2002). Biomedicine, then, is characterized by extensive reliance on collaboration among many parties, including universities, research institutes, new biotechnology firms, and mature pharmaceutical and chemical corporations (Arora and Gambardella 1994a, Lerner and Merges 1998, Stuart *et al.* 1999, Arora *et al.* 2001). Starting from the mid-1970s, the division of innovative labor has grown exponentially.

Figure IV.3 reveals that the number of inventors, assignees and backward citations per patent, as well as the number of licensing agreements and other collaborative agreements have soared. The number of researchers and research organizations involved in any single R&D activity has also increased. All in all, these phenomena reveal an increase in the complexity (and the cost) associated with the organization of R&D activities in pharmaceuticals.

---

[4] Rare diseases provide lower expected returns; nonetheless they have a higher probability of success.

Figure IV.3   The division of innovative labor in pharmaceutical R&D, 1976-2004

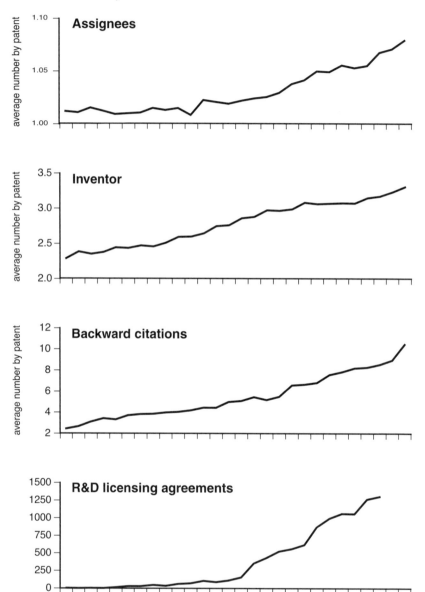

Source: our computations on Databiotech.com

IV.2   Some Plausible Explanations for the R&D Productivity Slowdown

As observed in the previous sections, although public and private R&D expenditures have grown exponentially, the number of new molecular entities appears to be substantially stable, leading to a decrease of TFP growth (see Chapter II). How to account for this puzzling evidence?

The decrease in R&D productivity can be explained by arguing that innovation is getting harder. Even if it is certainly possible that the life science innovation system is becoming increasingly more efficient, in a fashion analogous to Isaac Newton's famous remark about *standing on the shoulders of giants*, it is also possible that it is becoming increasingly difficult to discover new drugs, as the most obvious ideas are discovered first and the threshold for new discoveries rises. In the economic literature, articulated views of why innovation may be getting harder have focused on an innovation exhaustion argument or "fishing out" effect (Kortum, 1997; Segerstrom, 1998; Evenson 1991; Henderson and Cockburn, 1996; Cockburn, 2004; Jones, 2005). If new molecular entities are increasingly difficult to obtain, a growing number of researchers is needed to produce a constant number of innovative drugs, which in turn may lead to a constant rate of growth.

In other words, as long as difficulty is increasing over time, the research efforts should rise in order to obtain a constant flow of new inventions. The growth in research effort produces constant productivity growth if the size distribution of inventions is stationary. A key implication of this view is that the market value of inventions should rises over time (Kortum, 1997). The same is true if we assume that companies engage in R&D in order to enhance the quality of products. Firms that innovate and successfully launch patented drugs become industry leaders and earn temporary monopoly profits as a reward for their R&D efforts. Due to the growth in the population and in medical needs, the reward for innovation grows over time. However, counterbalancing this, innovating becomes progressively more difficult to obtain. As a result, the instantaneous probability of an innovation is constant along the balanced-growth path of the pharmaceutical sector despite the increase of R&D expenditures over time.

Therefore, the evidence presented so far can be accounted for by the burden of knowledge, specialization and division of labor. If knowledge accumulates as technology progresses, companies face an increasing knowledge burden. Innovators can compensate in their search strategies by seeking narrower expertise, with implications for the organization of innovative activity: a greater reliance on networks of R&D collaborations and division of labor among large pharmaceutical companies and dedicated biotech firms (DBFs). The growing complexity of biomedical research exerts a negative effect on long-run economic growth unless some paradigmatic shift resets and simplifies the knowledge space, causing a fall in the burden of knowledge. To increase the long-run growth rate, a technological shift must actually change the shape of the idea production function, so that newer and better ideas are somehow obtained more easily (Romer, 1990; Grossman and Helpman, 1991; Aghion and Howitt, 1992; Jones 2004).

Indeed, the decoding of the human genome as well as advances in information technology could lead to an upward shift in the production function for ideas. General-purpose technologies (GPTs) are technologies able to change permanently the production function for ideas (see Helpman, 1998). According to Bresnahan and Trajtenberg (1996), GPTs should have the following three characteristics:

1. *Pervasiveness:* the GPT should spread to many areas of application;

2. *Improvement:* the GPT should get better over time and, hence, should keep lowering the costs of its users;

3. *Innovation spawning:* the GPT should make it easier to invent and produce new products or processes.

The third property is by far the most important. Griliches (1957) for instance explains why hybrid corn was not an invention immediately adaptable everywhere, but was rather an invention of a method of inventing, a method of breeding superior corn for specific localities and similar considerations have been applied to the invention of PCR at Cetus (Rabinow, 1997). Theoretical models predict that at the arrival of GPTs (Jovanovic and Rousseau, 2005):

1. Productivity should slow down;

2. The cost of skilled labor should rise compared to those of the unskilled;

3. Entry, exit, mergers and acquisitions should rise;

4. Stock prices should initially fall if the advent of the new GPT was sudden and unforeseen and the old capital is not essential for the production of the new one. If these conditions hold, new and small companies should outperform old ones;

5. In an open economy, GPTs should cause the trade balance to worsen.

As David (1991) has pointed out, a GPT does not deliver productivity gains immediately upon arrival but requires complementary organizational revolutions. These were crucial, for instance, in order to relax some of the constraints to productivity growth associated with electrification and information technologies. This could explain why the promise of genomics in drug discovery, which was eagerly embraced in the 1990s, has not yet been fulfilled. Consequently, productivity slowdown could be related to the advent of platform technologies such as genomics, proteomics, high throughput screening and bioinformatics. The investment in GPTs will increase the time lag between the outlay of an R&D investment and the beginning of the associated revenue stream. This lag consists of two parts: a mean lag between project inception and completion (gestation lag), and the time from project completion to commercial application (application lag).[5] The gestation lag is particularly long in pharmaceuticals. In fact, DiMasi *et al.* (1994) estimate the lag from synthesis to approval of new drugs in the 1970s, 1980s and early 1990s and find that it averaged about twelve, fourteen and fifteen years, respectively. Toole (2000) estimates that a one percent increase in the stock of basic pharmaceutical research leads to an increase of 2.0 to 2.4 percent in the number of commercially available NMEs, after an average lag between additions to the stock of public basic research and commercialization of NMEs that is in the range of seventeen to nineteen years. In this con-

---

[5] Ravenscraft and Scherer (1982) regress deflated gross profits on a distributed lag of deflated R&D outlays and other variables and conclude that there is strong evidence that the lag structure is roughly bell-shaped, with a mean lag of from four to six years. More recently, Rouvinen (2002) comes to a similar conclusion based on OECD data stressing the high variability of the R&D-TFP relationship both in terms of timing and magnitude that might be associated with periods of structural change.

text, it is possible to explain why we observe a slowing of the generation or diffusion of new drugs in presence of increasing total factor
productivity (TFP) both in U.S. and in the EU (Chapter II). In sum,
as Rouvinen (2002) points out, the relationship between TFP and
R&D is not simultaneous, but the effects of inventor activities tend to
be produced with a time lag on general technological progress. The
time lag is not fixed and the recent decrease of TFP growth in the
U.S. could derive from a longer gestation lag needed in order to reap
the fruits of (post)-genomics GPTs.

Many scholars have investigated the connection between R&D
spending and productivity growth. Although economics has yet to
explain fully the determinants of TFP growth, even a cursory glance at
the empirical literature suggests that R&D plays an important role.[6]

Let A denote the knowledge capital. The change in A is given by
some production function W:

$$\dot{A} = W(R, A)$$

Where R represents R&D expenditures at a given time. Typically W
is increasing in the first argument and either increasing or decreasing
in the second one. If $\partial W / \partial A > 0$, past inventions raise the productivity
of research today. On the other hand, if the best inventions come first,
W is decreasing in A. As described in the box "Growth Decomposition
and TFP" in Chapter I, the pharmaceutical output is produced by
using the stock of knowledge and usual factors of production. Following Romer (1990) we have assumed that the production function is
increasing in each of its arguments with constant returns to capital
and labor and increasing returns to scale overall. In particular, by
using a Cobb-Douglas specification for both the final goods and
research technologies and switching to continuous time, we obtain a
generalized version of Romer's (1990) endogenous growth model:

$$Y = A_t^\alpha K_t^\alpha L_t^{1-\alpha}$$

where L is labor input and K is the aggregated capital stock as in
Equation [1] of box "Growth Decomposition and TFP".

---

[6] However, regardless of what functional form or estimating technique is used to identify
the contribution of R&D to TFP and hence to productivity growth, it has to be clear that
all available measures of R&D input and output are only imperfect proxies of innovation.

Suppose now, as in Jones and Williams (1997) that the R&D production function [1] takes the form:

$$\dot{A} = \sigma \frac{R^\lambda A^\phi}{(1+\psi)},$$

where σ is the productivity of R&D efforts. The presence of $0 \le \lambda \le 1$ may reflect duplication of effort in the research process, i.e. the social marginal product of R may be less than the private marginal product due to congestion externalities and duplication of R&D efforts. The parameter ϕ measures the net effect of knowledge spillovers. If the net effect is such that $\phi > 0$ we call this the *standing on shoulders effect* as the social returns to the knowledge stock is positive. On the contrary, if $\phi < 0$ it becomes increasingly difficult to discover new drugs, as the most obvious ideas are discovered first (the *fishing out effect*). A third distortion in the research process, highlighted by Grossman and Helpman (1991) and Aghion and Howitt (1992) is associated with creative destruction that is new drugs may replace old drugs: ψ follow-on drugs are produced that replace first in class products.

The traditional approach to estimate the effect of R&D expenditures on productivity is to treat R&D investment simply as an alternative capital investment. The R&D stock is included in the production function and the partial derivative of output with respect to that stock is treated as the rate of return to R&D.

The basic relationship is described by the following system of equations:

$$Y = e^{\mu t} Z^\xi K^\alpha L^{1-\alpha}$$

where Z is the R&D stock and we assume no depreciation of R&D capital. By standard growth accounting logic estimated TFP growth is given by:

$$\Delta \log \text{TFP} = \mu + \tilde{r} \frac{R}{Y} + \varepsilon$$

where R/Y is the R&D share of output and $\tilde{r}$ is the marginal productivity of R&D.

Indeed, the outcome of pharmaceutical R&D is an improvement in drug quality both in terms of completely NMEs and in terms of improvements of existing drugs. In order to capture quality effects, hedonic price indexes ought to be applied. As a result, more of a given increase in nominal sales will be classified as an increase in real output rather than as an increase in price and the rate of TFP growth will be higher. High tech industries such as the IT sector have shown higher productivity growth as statistical agencies have replaced regular price indexes with hedonic indexes. Similar considerations apply to pharmaceuticals. Passing to consider R&D inputs it has to be noted that R&D capital, which is typically calculated by cumulating past R&D investments, is largely intangible and has no market counterpart. Therefore, the economic value of the body of knowledge of companies, industries and nations is hard to measure. Moreover, as already noticed, knowledge does not deteriorate with age in the same manner that other capital assets do. Hence, the depreciation of the R&D capital is tightly related to the market value of new drugs that will diminish in time because of competition and regulation. Another measurement issue is related to potential inconsistency among the variables used to decompose the contribution of different production factors (capital, labor and knowledge). In most cases, it is impossible to remove from labor and capital inputs the labor and capital used to produce R&D. Therefore, part of U.S. capital accumulation and higher labor costs (see Chapter II) might be due to investments in R&D infrastructures and skilled human capital.

Finally, the effect of R&D spillovers and market for technologies has to be taken into account. In fact, firms benefit in many cases from R&D undertaken by other firms in the same industry or by firms in other industries or other countries, as well as from basic research performed in academic settings. A significant number of studies point to sizable spillover effects at the firm and industry levels. These effects are also present and likely to grow rapidly among firms in different countries: social rates of return from R&D remain significantly above private ones. Consequently, changes in the IPR regime and in the structure of the division of innovative labor at the international level would deeply affect productivity differentials among nations and technological transfer.

IV.3   Global Competition in Pharmaceutical R&D

Herein we analyze the locus of innovation in the pharmaceutical industry. Relying upon fine-grained information about R&D activities and launch of new products, we characterize the innovativeness of firms.

Table IV.2 shows the trends in R&D spending undertaken by the public and corporate sector for the period 1981-2002. Since the beginning of the 1980s, the amount of resources allocated to pharmaceutical R&D has significantly increased in all OECD countries both in absolute terms and relative to total public and private resources.

The U.S. ranks first in terms of total public and private R&D as well as public and private R&D intensity. Nevertheless, while Japan appears far below the U.S. benchmark, R&D effort of the EU-15 private companies is close enough to U.S. competitors. In 1996-2002, U.S. pharmaceutical companies' R&D intensity was 11.3 percent (9.8 percent in the first half of the 1980s), versus 10.04 percent (6.6 percent in 1981-1985) of European counterparts. Among European countries, northern countries (United Kingdom, Sweden, Denmark and Belgium) had the highest levels of private R&D intensity, also higher than the U.S. figure in 1996-2002.

These data have to be interpreted with extreme caution because several factors frustrate accurate accounting, such as the evaluation of R&D capital assets depreciation, the length of drug development projects, international differences in R&D statistics and so on. Moreover, global pharmaceutical players spend a significant share of their R&D budgets abroad. In Table IV.2, R&D expenditure and production are considered by location of the firm, but we do not distinguish the nationality of holding companies. Thus, if a corporation based in the U.S. devotes financial resources to R&D through its European branches, these flows are recorded as R&D undertaken in Europe, and vice versa. Indeed, looking at the BEA data for 2003, R&D performed by U.S. affiliates in all countries[7] amounts to $4.666 billion, whereas the figure for R&D performed by European affiliates in the U.S. is higher and amounts to $7.679 billion.

---

[7] Data for the R&D performed by U.S. affiliates in Europe is only available for the year 1999 and it equals to $2.575 billion (72 percent of the worldwide figure).

Table IV.2   Annual private and public pharmaceutical R&D expenditures (€ millions, PPP) as a percentage of total pharmaceutical production value (private) and national healthcare budget (public)[1]

		1981-85		1986-90		1991-95		1996-02	
		€m	%*	€m	%*	€m	%*	€m	%*
Belgium	private	145	11.76	220	11.96	330	10.59	637	11.39
	public	–	–	–	–	–	–	–	–
France	private	543	5.32	882	6.07	1,736	8.43	2,594	8.99
	public	892	1.84	1,436	2.11	1,712	2.10	2,388	2.25
Germany	private	718	9.35	1,168	10.85	1,211	7.83	2,012	9.43
	public	224	0.38	281	0.37	1,800	1.32	2,240	1.33
Sweden	private	130	16.22	264	20.90	513	19.93	1,087	21.89
	public	216	2.42	249	2.30	299	2.40	–	–
Denmark	private	53	9.35	107	12.28	196	14.46	454	16.55
	public	79	1.47	109	1.80	209	2.78	254	2.50
Italy	private	444	3.66	783	5.20	694	3.99	610	2.83
	public	–	–	260	0.46	238	0.36	181	0.23
Spain	private	63	1.55	143	2.60	236	2.94	402	3.89
	public	13	0.09	83	0.40	120	0.37	176	0.42
UK	private	758	12.10	1,494	16.04	2,573	18.26	4,095	22.00
	public	–	–	–	–	1,424	2.15	1,402	1.97
EU-15	private	2,823	6.62	4,995	8.21	7,779	11.05	12,016	10.04
	public	686	0.72	1,120	0.69	4,521	1.20	5,552	1.01
U.S.	private	2,634	9.83	4,995	11.22	8,800	12.50	11,621	11.29
	public	6,399	4.53	9,999	4.51	14,272	3.79	23,341	4.24
Canada	private	–	–	134	4.70	285	7.40	516	9.69
	public	181	0.86	293	0.96	409	0.98	1,017	1.96
Japan	private	1,318	6.49	2,161	7.59	3,431	9.51	4,721	10.49
	public	2,174	3.32	2,944	3.17	4,091	3.01	4,990	2.89

*Private R&D expenditures as a percentage of the value of pharmaceutical production; public R&D disbursements as a percentage of total public healthcare expenditures.

(1) R&D data are missing for Austria, Greece, Luxembourg, and Portugal for the whole period; for Belgium in the years 1990 and 1991; for Denmark and Ireland in the year 2000 and for Sweden in the year 2002. Production data are missing for Luxembourg and Ireland (whole period) and Germany (1987-1990). Shares of production are obtained as weighted average from available data

Source: OECD, ANBERD Database and STAN Database (latest data available)

Despite limitations in terms of international comparability among nationalities of the corporations involved in the research activities, the U.S. is the country where the largest R&D expenditure is carried out. In this respect the role of public R&D activities are much higher than in the EU-25. The share of R&D in national health care budgets was 4.24 percent in the U.S. and 1.01 percent in EU-15 countries over the period 1996-2002.

Besides R&D expenditures, the empirical literature aimed at measuring technological change has proposed a wide set of measures and indicators to evaluate R&D outcomes. Among them, the most prominent are patent-based indicators.

Patents are a unique source of information about innovative activities, particularly in the pharmaceutical industry, where they play an important role in protecting returns from R&D (see Cohen *et al.*, 2000).

We analyze all pharmaceutical and biotechnological patents granted from 1974 to 2005 by the United States Patent and Trademark Office (USPTO) to inventors and institutions located in the U.S., Japan, and Europe.[8]

Table IV.3 reports the share of USPTO patents granted within the pharmaceutical domain to inventors and assignees classified according to their location.

All available evidence on R&D outcomes shows that the U.S. is the main locus of innovative activities, and its leadership has strengthened over time.

Table IV.3 testifies that the majority of patents in pharmaceuticals are held by inventors located in the U.S.[9] The number of pharmaceutical patents held by U.S.-based inventors increased by five percentage points between 1986-1995 and 1996-2005. The increase is even more striking if we weight each patent by its importance, as measured by the number of citations it receives (see Table IV.4). Canada, Denmark and Sweden are the only other countries that have experienced an increase in the

---

[8] Pharmaceutical patents have been identified based on the International Patent Classification. Specifically, we have selected patents in classes A61K (preparations for medical, dental, or toilet purposes) and A01N (preservation of bodies of humans or animals or parts thereof). See Lanjouw and Cockburn (2001).

[9] Patents granted by the U.S. Patent and Trademark Office might "overestimate" the patenting performance of U.S. scientists and research organizations as compared to foreign ones. Dernis and Khan (2004) estimates that the share of USPTO patents of U.S. companies in 1999 (52.6 percent) is well above their share of EPO patents (27.8 percent) and triadic patent families (34 percent). However, this problem may be attenuated by comparing patent shares over time and by using multiple indicators of innovation and R&D performances.

Table IV.3   Shares of USPTO-granted pharmaceutical patents by nationality of the assignee (A) and location of the inventor (I)

	1976-1985			1986-1995			1996-2005		
	A	I	I-A	A	I	I-A	A	I	I-A
France	5.88	5.84	-0.03	5.31	5.31	-0.01	5.64	5.73	0.09
Germany	11.29	11.47	0.18	9.58	9.71	0.12	7.19	7.29	0.10
Sweden	0.78	0.81	0.03	0.73	0.72	0.00	1.24	1.13	-0.10
Denmark	0.31	0.32	0.00	0.58	0.60	0.02	0.84	0.87	0.02
Italy	2.12	2.26	0.14	2.21	2.47	0.26	1.30	1.66	0.36
Spain	0.16	0.16	0.00	0.28	0.33	0.06	0.31	0.39	0.08
UK	5.76	7.72	1.96	4.44	5.99	1.56	3.68	5.02	1.34
Other EU-15	1.37	1.79	0.42	2.26	2.04	-0.22	2.52	2.25	-0.27
New EU States	0.91	0.91	0.00	0.89	0.91	0.02	0.24	0.35	0.11
EU-25	28.59	31.29	2.70	26.28	28.09	1.81	22.96	24.70	1.74
U.S.	57.57	50.88	-6.69	55.92	52.02	-3.90	60.06	57.35	-2.71
Canada	0.74	1.24	0.50	1.26	1.53	0.27	2.67	2.79	0.12
Japan	10.31	10.48	0.17	13.32	13.44	0.12	8.47	8.71	0.24
Switzerland	1.51	4.20	2.69	1.26	2.54	1.28	1.46	1.41	-0.05
Other	1.27	1.92	0.64	1.96	2.38	0.43	4.38	5.04	0.66

Source: our computations on USPTO data (granted patents only)

share of pharmaceutical patents granted to locally based inventors between those two periods, although the increase is much lower than in the U.S. In addition, the residual category "Other" has experienced a strong increase in the share of patents and citations. Within this category, the largest share of patents (in terms of both inventors and assignees) is owned by Israel, Australia, Republic of Korea, India, Taiwan and China. Among them, India, Korea, and China have experienced the fastest growth.[10]

The location of the inventor can be considered a good proxy of the location of the research activities, pointing to a larger share of research undertaken by U.S. inventors, increasing over time. More in general, results in Table IV.4 confirm that U.S. institutions outperform EU counterparts in attracting high quality human capital and/or in increasing the productivity of talents they employ.

---

[10] This trend will be further explored below in the section devoted to discuss the role of the emerging economies in the innovation process in pharmaceuticals.

Table IV.4   Shares of patent citations of USPTO-granted pharmaceutical patents by nationality of the assignee (A) and location of the inventor (I)

	1976-1985			1986-1995			1996-2005		
	A	I	I-A	A	I	I-A	A	I	I-A
France	4.73	4.84	*0.11*	3.92	4.08	*0.15*	4.54	4.87	*0.33*
Germany	8.16	8.32	*0.16*	6.13	6.29	*0.16*	4.94	5.13	*0.19*
Sweden	1.23	1.19	*-0.04*	0.75	0.71	*-0.04*	1.24	1.19	*-0.05*
Denmark	0.35	0.37	*0.02*	0.53	0.59	*0.06*	0.48	0.48	*0.00*
Italy	1.14	1.27	*0.14*	1.28	1.46	*0.18*	0.74	1.15	*0.41*
Spain	0.09	0.09	*0.00*	0.14	0.16	*0.02*	0.14	0.21	*0.07*
UK	5.13	6.94	*1.81*	3.48	5.03	*1.55*	3.76	4.85	*1.09*
Other EU-15	1.34	1.65	*0.31*	2.06	1.65	*-0.42*	1.98	1.55	*-0.43*
New EU States	0.60	0.64	*0.04*	0.38	0.42	*0.04*	0.11	0.23	*0.12*
EU-25	22.78	25.32	*2.55*	18.68	20.40	*1.71*	17.92	19.66	*1.74*
U.S.	64.35	59.10	*-5.25*	67.83	64.62	*-3.20*	70.66	68.18	*-2.48*
Canada	1.15	1.63	*0.49*	1.47	1.88	*0.41*	2.30	2.43	*0.13*
Japan	9.48	9.55	*0.07*	9.11	9.18	*0.08*	5.34	5.50	*0.17*
Switzerland	1.12	2.75	*1.63*	1.25	1.95	*0.70*	1.08	1.09	*0.01*
Other	1.13	1.65	*0.52*	1.66	1.97	*0.30*	2.70	3.14	*0.43*

Source: our computations on USPTO data (granted patents only)

Interestingly enough, the share of EU-25 inventors is higher than the share of EU-25 institutional assignees. The opposite is true for the U.S., even if the imbalance is gradually fading away. In other words, there are more European inventors involved into research assigned to U.S. organizations than *vice-versa*, although the globalization of R&D activities is eroding this disparity.

Indeed, the "brain drain" from Europe towards the U.S. is increasing. About 50 percent of all Europeans completing a Ph.D. in the U.S. stay on for longer periods afterwards, and many of them stay permanently (Finn, 2003). The U.S. Department of Labor statistics show that over half of European Ph.D. students in Science and Engineering graduating in the U.S. in the period 1988-95 are still in the U.S. even 5 years after graduation (Johnson & Regets, 1998). The most important reasons keeping European scientists and engineers abroad relate to the quality of work. Better prospects and projects and easier access to leading technologies were most often cited as reasons behind plans to work abroad.[11]

Historically, the biotechnology revolution took place in the U.S., star scientists still work there and even today the U.S. is more specialized in biotechnology than the European countries. With the single exception of Denmark, with the highest specialization in the biotechnology sector,[12] on average European countries and Japan tend to be more focused on non-biological pharmaceutical patents. As will be shown later in this chapter, the U.S. industry is characterized by a wider division of innovative labor than Europe, where dedicated biotechnology firms effectively connect the research undertaken within universities and research laboratories to industrial applications. With few exceptions, the raise of the biotechnology sector is neither a European nor a Japanese phenomenon. As for the emerging economies, OECD data report a high specialization index for India and China, close to the U.S. value.

Finally, we look at innovative output as measured by the number of New Molecular Entities (NMEs) launched since 1994. We have already pointed out the fact that the number of NMEs introduced worldwide has remained substantially stable over the 1990s, sharply decreasing in the years 2000-2003 and stable afterwards, despite an exponential growth trend in the R&D expenditures (see Figure IV.1 and Table IV.2). In this scenario of decreasing returns to R&D investments, U.S. multinationals are still worldwide leaders in terms of number and sales of NMEs, confirming the trend detected in GOP (2000).

Table IV.5 reports the number of NMEs launched worldwide, by nationality of the R&D corporation, over the period 1994-2005. Since nominal values experience large fluctuations, the share of NMEs is computed considering three-year moving average, to highlight global trends.[13] The largest share of NMEs was introduced by U.S. corporations (37 percent over the period 1994-2004, and 53.3 percent in 2005).

---

[11] For more details and statistics on the European brain drain phenomenon, see MERIT (2003).

[12] The Danish profile of specialization is driven by non-medical biotechnologies. See OECD Biotechnology Statistics (2006).

[13] The exception being the year 2005, where the share is computed considering only 2005 values.

Table IV.5   Number of New Molecular Entities launched, by nationality of R&D corporation, 1994-2005[1]

		'94	'95	'96	'97	'98	'99	'00	'01	'02	'03	'04	'05
U.S.	Num	12	14	14	19	22	17	14	18	13	13	10	16
	% (MA3)	–	30.3	33.3	39.3	41.1	41.1	40.2	40.2	42.7	37.1	42.9	53.3*
EU-15	Num	9	13	18	18	11	14	14	5	10	4	11	3
	% (MA3)	–	30.3	34.8	33.6	30.5	30.2	27.0	25.9	18.4	25.8	19.8	10.0*
Japan	Num	18	10	6	9	5	10	7	5	10	3	5	5
	% (MA3)	–	25.8	17.7	14.3	17.0	17.1	18.0	19.6	17.5	18.6	14.3	16.7*
Other	Num	3	8	7	5	6	5	4	9	3	10	5	6
	% (MA3)	–	13.7	14.2	12.9	11.3	11.6	14.7	14.3	21.4	18.6	23.1	20.0*
Total		42	45	45	51	44	46	39	37	36	30	31	30

(1) Based on the location of the headquarters. MA3: Three-years moving average.
*2005 shares have been computed considering 2005 values (not moving averages).

Source: IMS Health—World Review (various issues)

Table IV.6   Top 50 NMEs by nationality of the main marketing company, 1985-2002

Company Nationality[1]	Number of NMEs				sales (%)			
	'85-'89	'95-'99	'98-'02	'01-'05	'85-'89	'95-'99	'98-'02	'01-'05
U.S.	17	24	27	29	41.49	69.12	65.14	63.96
Japan	20	3	3	3	37.33	3.92	6.35	7.53
Switzerland	3	6	9	10	2.91	7.78	9.02	16.94
EU-15	10	16	11	8	18.28	18.54	19.49	11.58
UK	3	8	3	4	6.53	9.38	13.84	5.68
Germany	7	4	3	2	11.75	3.33	2.07	4.28
Netherlands	0	1	0	0	0.00	0.80	0.00	0.00
France	0	3	2	1	0.00	5.03	1.77	1.16
Belgium	0	0	1	1	0.00	0.00	0.75	0.46
Denmark	0	0	2	0	0.00	0.00	1.06	0.00

(1) Based on the location of the headquarters.

Source: IMS Health—World Review (various issues)

In the previous sections, we observed that the decline of R&D productivity hits mainly the U.S. pharmaceutical industry. However, U.S. companies still control more than half of sales of NMEs (see Table IV.6) and this trend is deemed to be reinforced by the growing availability of biopharmaceutical products (see Figure V.7). By looking jointly at the number of top 50 NMEs and their share of sales of EU-15 and U.S. corporations, data suggest that the European companies are experiencing a competitive disadvantage in selling their new drugs. Indeed, while the number of NMEs introduced by U.S. corporations from 2001 to 2005 is 3.6 times larger than the number of NMEs introduced by EU-15 corporations, sales figures are 5.5 times larger. Put differently, the average market share of NME introduced by U.S. corporations is 2.2 percent, as compared to 1.4 percent for European companies. After a steep decline in the second half of the 1990s, Japanese companies have regained part of their market share of NME in 2001-2005, moving from 3.9 percent to 7.5 percent.

Whereas European companies have an increasing share of their total sales from newly introduced products, the reverse is true for U.S. companies (see Table IV.7). At the end of the 1990s, the product portfolio of U.S. corporations had a higher share of total sales from newly launched products. In other words, the products of European multinationals tended to be older as compared to U.S. counterparts. The share of total 1997 sales from products launched since 1988 was equal to 32 percent for U.S. corporations, against 16 percent of EU-15 corporations. Starting from 2001, the U.S. and EU-15 has inverted their positions. The share of sales from newly introduced products has increased for EU-15 corporations to 26 percent, while it has decreased to 22 percent for U.S. corporations. The portfolio of the top Swiss companies (in terms of 2005 sales of newly introduced products) is the youngest, with newly introduced products accounting for 29 percent of sales.

The role of Emerging Economies

Here we expand our view to take into consideration the role played by developing countries. Among them, India and China are strengthening their position in the pharmaceutical industry as evidenced by the significant increase in their share of pharmaceutical patents and publications. The emergence of new Asian competitors has important implications for the European pharmaceutical industry. As long as the process of harmonization of China and India in the international context will be completed, the comparative advantages of Europe could be vulnerable to the competition of these emerging economies characterized by growing human capital and demand for pharmaceuticals.

Table IV.7   Contribution to total sales from new products

Company Nationality[1]	% of total 1997 sales[2] from products launched since 1988	% of total 2002 sales[3] from products launched since 1998	% of total 2005 sales[3] from products launched since 2001
U.S.	32	28	22
Japan	29	30	16
Switzerland	14	29	29
EU-15	16	23	26

(1) Based on the location of the headquarters. (2) Top 100 companies. (3) Top 50 companies.

Source: IMS Health—World Review (various issues)

Development of a domestic drug industry is a priority for countries such as China and India, which face a high portion of unmet medical needs, own a large internal market, a growing manufacturing industry and a high level of human capital and infrastructure for biopharmaceutical R&D. A big shake-up is occurring in the pharmaceutical sector of China, India, Brazil, South Africa and many other developing countries. In recent years[14] they have aligned their legislation with the provisions of the TRIPS agreement, entry into force of which is part of WTO obligations.[15] The enforcement of TRIPS represents a radical change in the IPR systems of those countries, and economic theory predicts an increase in the incentives of local producers to engage in R&D activities rather than relying on reverse-engineered products. This is particularly true in the pharmaceutical industry, where patents play a prominent role in protecting the returns from innovative activities (Mansfield, 1986; Levin *et al.*, 1987; Cohen *et al.*, 2000). In addition, the expansion of intellectual property rights is expected to favor investments from foreign multinationals, lured by the large markets and the low labor costs.[16]

---

[14] India and Egypt were among the last ones, amending their legislation in January 2005.

[15] TRIPS (Trade-Related Aspects of Intellectual Property Rights) are the IP agreements of the WTO covering everything from copyrights to trademarks, trade secrets and patents. Its provisions on pharmaceutical patents entered into force in January 1995 in developed countries. However, developing countries were given 10 more years (until January 2005) to adapt their legislation. For a recent and thorough analysis of the effect of the TRIPS agreement on the Indian pharmaceutical market see Chaudhuri *et al.* (2006).

[16] Although it is well-known that a serious intellectual property rights protection and a liberalized pharmaceutical market are necessary but not sufficient conditions, alone, for the creation of an internal R&D network (it depends on a sum of endogenous conditions varying from the organization of the university system to that of the public administration, to the efficacy and efficiency of the public spending), they surely represent important factors to stimulate the production of innovative drugs and, with it, the inflows of capital to sustain R&D projects.

Evidence of increased patenting activity following the TRIPS agreement, and also of increased research targeting developing countries needs (Lanjouw and Cockburn, 2001; Chadha, 2005) is available for India. A case study of four Indian pharmaceutical firms shows that Indian generic manufacturers have started to build basic R&D capabilities, pursuing different R&D and marketing strategies and also looking at examples from the software industry (Athreye and Kale, 2006).

India has experienced strong overall economic growth over the last 20 years, led by the development in the national software industry. Traditional factors are of little help in explaining the sustained growth either of the industry or the overall Indian economy: clusters, support by venture capitalists and government policies have played none or little role in the process (Arora and Gambardella, 2006). Rather, the root of the success of the Indian software industry can be traced back to labor cost advantages, abundant human capital (high number of trained engineers relative to domestic needs), diffuse knowledge of the English language, and entrepreneurship. Moreover, the Indian-born population in the U.S. has increased substantially over the 1990s, building strong business ties and diaspora networks in-between India and the U.S. and supplying India a flow of skill-enhanced return migration (Kapur, McHale, 2006). Saxenian (2005) reports that by 2000, over one-third of Silicon Valley's high-skilled workers were foreign-born, mainly from India and China.

These factors can potentially be applied to the development of the biopharmaceutical industry and so foster its growth. A good endowment in human capital is an important pre-condition for the sound development of such a research-intensive sector like pharmaceuticals. Since detailed datasets on the amount of researchers in the pharmaceutical sector are not available, in Table IV.8 we report the number of total resident researchers and their share of total employment in some OECD and developing countries. Even if the relative numbers for China and India are still far from the OECD level, the absolute numbers are really impressive. China already has the second largest number of researchers in the world, just behind the U.S., and graduates the most each year along with India (OECD, 2005).

Moreover, the share of researchers employed in the business sector shows that most human capital is devoted to activities directly aimed

Table IV.8   Number of researchers by country

Countries	total number of resident researchers (thousands)	resident researchers/ '000 employed	researchers employed in business enterprise as a % of total researchers
U.S. (2000)	1,261,227	8.6	80.5
EU-25 (2001)	1,117,361	5.6	52.1
China (2003)	862,108	1.0*	56.2
Japan (2003)	675,330	10.4	67.9
Russia (2003)	487,477	7.8*	54.9
India (1998)	95,428	1.0	36.6
Brazil (2001)	70,940	0.2	32.7
Taiwan (2001)	59,656	6.4	59.2
OECD countries (2000)	3,378,725	6.6	63.6

*2001.
Source: OECD—Science, Technology and Industry Scoreboard (2003, 2005).

at marketable innovations. Although R&D expenditure data show that the budget of a researcher in these countries is still considerably lower than for most advanced OECD economies, these differences are deemed to disappear in the near future, since some of these economies are rapidly catching up.[17]

Until recently, China was lagging behind in pharmaceutical research, with its companies being concentrated almost exclusively in the production of generic drugs for the home market: Chinese generic producers manage to reproduce and to bring onto the Chinese market 97.4 percent of the Western chemical entities sold in China. However, things are slowly changing, not only as an effect of the TRIPS agreement, but also due to a greater awareness by the government of the strategic importance of the pharmaceutical sector. Starting from 1992, China had already made substantial changes to its IP legislation, by recognizing product patents on pharmaceuticals and extending patent protection to 20 years. In the year 2002, other important modifications on licensing and infringement made Chinese legislation fully TRIPS compliant. Although Chinese entrepreneurs have been relatively slow in acknowledging the value of intellectual property, in such a way that its enforcement is weak, investments in R&D in this sector

[17] See OECD (2003a and 2003b).

are rapidly increasing in quality and quantity. Firms finance most R&D expenditure. Government financing of R&D is low but increasing. However, China can count on a vast pool of highly educated researchers at low cost; it is estimated that R&D in China costs only 30 percent of that in developed countries.

Table IV.9 shows that in the last decade, the U.S. share of biomedical scientific publications follows a downward trend. Since 1995, it has decreased by 7.5 percentage points. The European share has increased from 36.6 percent in 1995 to 39.0 in 2001 and been rather stable afterwards. The Japanese share has decreased more than two percentage points. The average annual growth in the number of publications is 6.8 percent for the EU-25 countries, versus 4.3 and 4.0 percent respectively for the U.S. and Japan. In comparison, Chinese publications have augmented at an average rate of 21.6 percent each year, and China has gained more than six percentage points in global share. Even though less pronounced than the Chinese increase, the share of biomedical scientific publications by Indian authors has increased from 0.8 percent in 1995 to 2.0 percent in 2005, with an average annual growth in the number of publications of 12.6 percent. South Africa and Israel have not substantially changed their shares, while the share of Brazil has increased from 0.8 percent in 1995 to 1.9 percent in 2005.

Table IV.10 reports the number of pharmaceutical and biotechnology patents granted by the patent offices in selected developing countries. Table IV.11 shows the patenting activity in the U.S. by assignees and inventors located in other selected countries. Data show that, in recent years, the number of patents in pharmaceuticals and biotechnology granted by the Chinese patent office has increased, as well as the count of U.S. patents granted to Chinese inventors (at an average annual rate of 22.5 and 17.6 percent respectively for the period 2000-2005). Taken together, these increases indicate a process of accumulation of scientific and technological capabilities. India's recent performance in biopharmaceutical innovation, as reflected in patents granted, is similar to the Chinese. India has taken longer than China to align its legislation with TRIPS provisions, having introduced product patents only at the beginning of 2005, more than thirty years after their abolition in 1970, in favor of considering effective only patents for manufacturing processes. The Indian Patent Act (1970) led

Table IV.9   Biomedical scientific publications by country: number (thousands), growth and share of total publications

		'95	'96	'97	'98	'99	'00	'01	'02	'03	'04	'05	Growth '95-'05[1]
China	no.	5.1	6.1	7.1	8.2	9.1	12.3	15.1	18.2	23.1	28.8	36.1	+21.6
	%	1.9	2.2	2.4	2.7	2.9	3.5	4.1	4.7	5.7	6.6	7.5	
India	no.	2.9	3.1	3.1	3.5	3.9	4.7	5.5	6.0	6.9	7.6	9.4	+12.6
	%	1.1	1.1	1.1	1.1	1.2	1.3	1.5	1.6	1.7	1.7	2.0	
Israel	no.	3.8	3.9	3.9	3.7	4.0	4.6	4.7	5.1	5.4	5.7	5.9	+4.6
	%	1.4	1.4	1.3	1.2	1.2	1.3	1.3	1.3	1.3	1.3	1.2	
Russia	no.	0.8	1.2	1.7	2.5	2.6	3.6	3.5	3.6	3.9	2.7	2.3	+10.3
	%	0.3	0.4	0.6	0.8	0.8	1.0	1.0	0.9	1.0	0.6	0.5	
S. Africa	no.	1.0	1.0	1.0	1.1	1.1	1.3	1.3	1.3	1.3	1.4	1.6	+5.0
	%	0.4	0.4	0.4	0.3	0.3	0.4	0.4	0.3	0.3	0.3	0.3	
Brazil	no.	2.1	2.3	2.7	3.1	3.7	4.4	4.9	5.9	6.8	7.8	8.9	+15.5
	%	0.8	0.8	0.9	1.0	1.2	1.2	1.3	1.5	1.7	1.8	1.9	
EU-25	no.	96.4	104.0	108.2	114.5	121.2	135.6	143.7	150.9	156.5	167.7	185.4	+6.8
	%	36.6	36.9	37.2	37.6	38.1	38.4	39.0	39.0	38.3	38.3	38.6	
U.S.	no.	123.6	130.8	133.3	135.2	138.7	149.9	153.0	157.9	165.9	176.9	189.1	+4.3
	%	46.9	46.5	45.8	44.4	43.7	42.4	41.5	40.8	40.6	40.4	39.4	
Japan	no.	27.9	29.3	29.8	32.5	33.5	37.2	37.1	37.9	38.6	39.3	41.1	+4.0
	%	10.6	10.4	10.2	10.7	10.5	10.5	10.1	9.8	9.5	9.0	8.6	
Total	%	263.6	281.6	290.8	304.3	317.7	353.4	368.7	386.8	408.5	437.8	479.8	+3.1

(1) Average annual percentage growth.

Source: PubMed.

to the birth of a thriving population of generic drug manufacturers that have become the world leading suppliers of generic drugs (Hoffman, 2005).

As far as industrial competitiveness is concerned, if these trends persist, China and India will consolidate their competitive positions, becoming attractive destinations for foreign direct investment by pharmaceutical multinational corporations. These countries provide a serious threat to the role of the European pharmaceutical industry, diverting the vertical "resource seeking" foreign direct investment of U.S. companies. U.S. companies are looking for locations where it is possible to reproduce or better the productivity conditions of their home country (specifically, the high labor productivity thanks to the high capital/labor ratio) but with a lower cost of production factors.

Table IV.10   Patents in pharmaceuticals and biotechnology, selected patent offices (1995-2005)

		'95	'96	'97	'98	'99	'00	'01	'02	'03	'04	'05
China	no.	2,682	2,905	3,501	4,057	4,392	6,891	9,010	9,947	11,155	12,805	19,017
	% change	–	8.3	20.5	15.9	8.3	56.9	30.8	10.4	12.1	14.8	48.5
Russia	no.	1,026	810	1,395	1,420	1,449	1,442	940	1,491	2,066	2,893	3,708
	% change	–	-21.1	72.2	1.8	2.0	-0.5	-34.8	58.6	38.6	40.0	28.2
Brazil	no.	415	398	913	724	1,844	2,871	2,027	1,894	1,492	2,589	2,456
	% change											
South Africa	no.	1,138	1,390	1,345	1,405	1,272	508	460	1,265	1,380	1,520	1,224
	% change		22.1	-3.2	4.5	-9.5	-60.1	-9.4	175.0	9.1	10.1	-19.5
Israel	no.	703	693	323	534	773	602	1,259	1,364	679	754	987
	% change		-1.4	-53.4	65.3	44.8	-22.1	109.1	8.3	-50.2	11.0	30.9
India	no.	68	80	173	107	172	198	194	217	310	123	–
	% change		17.6	116.3	-38.2	60.7	15.1	-2.0	11.9	42.9	-60.3	–

Source: our computations on Databiotech.com.

Table IV.11   USPTO patents assigned to institutions and invented by researchers in selected emerging countries

	Patents Assignee (A)			Patents Invented (I)			I-A		
	2000	2005	growth	2000	2005	growth	2000	2005	growth
Israel	461	778	68.8%	742	1,184	59.6%	281	406	44.5%
India	71	333	369.0%	230	554	140.9%	159	221	39.0%
China	34	96	182.4%	127	286	125.2%	93	190	104.3%
South Africa	29	42	44.8%	92	122	32.6%	63	80	27.0%
Russia	21	36	71.4%	96	181	88.5%	75	145	93.3%
Brazil	10	30	200.0%	62	126	103.2%	52	96	84.6%

Source: our computations on Databiotech.com.

As for scientific leadership in the life sciences, the 2000 Lisbon Agenda to make the EU the most competitive and innovative hub in the world is extremely unrealistic. The U.S. system is still pre-eminent and there is little chance that Europe will ever supersede it. Maybe China will, as a growing number of high-tech companies have been relocating their R&D facilities to China, as well as India. As a result, in 2004 there were already over six hundred research facilities from multinational corporations in China, including all the most important pharmaceutical MNCs.

IV.4 The International System of Division of Innovative Labor

Structural breakthroughs in the pharmaceutical industry over the last two decades, mainly driven by technological and institutional shocks, have had a major impact on firms' organization of innovative activities (Orsenigo *et al.*, 2001; Powell, Koput, Smith-Doer, 1996). As a result, the pharmaceutical industry has been increasingly conceived as a system or network. Innovative activities, but also the production and commercialization of drugs, rests with and involves, either directly or indirectly, a large variety of actors endowed with complementary resources and capabilities tied together by a system of division of innovative labor. Consequently, looking at individual firms only provides a partial picture of the competitiveness and innovativeness of the industry. The dynamic interactions among all the actors involved in the innovation process need to be considered.

Patent co-inventorship is a strong form of collaboration, involving direct contact and sharing of ideas among inventors. Therefore, the share of co-invented patents involving inventors located in different countries is a good proxy of the degree of internationalization of the innovation process in the life sciences.

Table IV.12 shows some relevant statistics on co-invented patents, as a measure of the extent of internationalization of the innovation process in the life sciences.

The results in Table IV.12 show that pharmaceutical R&D is increasingly globalized (i.e., the share of co-invented patents involving inventors located in a single region is decreasing). The U.S. research system occupies a prominent position in the international network of division of innovative labor.

U.S. dominance appears even stronger when we consider patent citations data. Table IV.13 suggests that patents assigned to U.S. institutions have a much greater impact on future innovative activity. U.S. biopharmaceutical patents received 6.07 citations on average between 1996 and 2005, far more than European (3.18) and Japanese (2.12) ones. Furthermore, the largest share (almost half) of the European and Japanese citations go to U.S. patents, although this finding must be interpreted with caution, since we are considering data on patents granted by the USPTO. Nevertheless, the trends in the EU to U.S.

Table IV.12   The internationalization of R&D activities: co-invented patents

		1976-1985	1986-1995	1996-2005
		U.S.		
Patent count		9,599	16,401	36,328
Mean number of inventors		1.80	2.35	2.54
Share of co-invented patents		51.82%	68.11%	65.26%
of which:	**U.S.-U.S.**	96.20%	93.60%	90.66%
	U.S.-EU	2.90%	4.87%	8.02%
	U.S.-JP	0.92%	1.62%	1.46%
		EU-25		
Patent count		5,993	9,086	16,557
Mean number of inventors		2.89	3.45	3.11
Share of co-invented patents		79.84%	84.66%	72.78%
of which: [1]	**EU-EU**	96.82%	92.45%	83.28%
	EU-U.S.	3.01%	7.07%	15.78%
	EU-JP	0.19%	0.61%	1.22%
		Japan		
Patent count		1,975	4,208	5,537
Mean number of inventors		4.04	4.30	3.66
Share of co-invented patents		92.51%	93.49%	79.19%
of which: [1]	**JP-JP**	97.04%	94.46%	89.51%
	JP-U.S.	2.52%	4.60%	7.91%
	JP-EU	0.49%	1.19%	3.35%

(1) Percentage do not sum to 100 because the inventors of a patent may have located in more than two countries. Source: our computations on USPTO data (granted patents only)

and Japan to U.S. pattern of citations reveal the increasing importance of U.S. research for inventors located in Europe and Japan.

Table IV.14 shows the evolution of R&D collaborations since 1991, by location of the company that originated/developed the innovation. The number of licensing agreements has increased from 2,257 in 1991-1997 to 3,528 in the period 1998-2004. The Table shows that U.S. institutions play a pivotal role in the international network of R&D and marketing licensing agreements. Besides being the most prolific in terms of licensing agreements, U.S. institutions are also the main partners of licensing agreements by EU companies and organizations, both as licensors and licensees. EU institutions play a subordinate role, as reflected in the much smaller number of agreements in

**Table IV.13 The internationalization of R&D activities:
patent citations**

		1976-1985	1986-1995	1996-2005
		U.S.		
Patent count		9,599	16,401	36,328
Number of citations[1]		10,131	52,694	220,371
Mean number of citations		1.06	3.21	6.07
of which:[2]	U.S.- >U.S.	72.35%	70.48%	70.32%
	U.S.- >EU	18.74%	18.37%	18.80%
	U.S.- >JP	5.22%	7.15%	6.60%
		EU-25		
Patent count		5,993	9,086	16,557
Number of citations[1]		4,849	17,782	52,689
Mean number of citations		0.81	1.96	3.18
of which:[2]	EU- >EU	55.56%	49.22%	42.96%
	EU- >U.S.	35.39%	39.74%	49.09%
	EU- >JP	5.40%	8.43%	7.37%
		Japan		
Patent count		1,975	4,208	5,537
Number of citations[1]		1,525	7,046	11,730
Mean number of citations		0.77	1.67	2.12
of which:[2]	JP- >JP	40.98%	35.99%	35.89%
	JP- >U.S.	35.08%	37.82%	41.61%
	JP- >EU	21.57%	23.97%	21.99%

(1) Only backward citations to pharmaceutical patents are considered. (2) Percentage do not sum
to 100 because patent inventors may have located in more than two countries.

Source: our computations on USPTO data (granted patents only)

which they are involved. The relatively low number of intra-EU
agreements confirms the secondary role of the EU in pharmaceutical
R&D.

Despite the increasing globalization of the pharmaceutical industry
described in Chapter III (Section 5) and even though the international
licensing deals are increasing in absolute terms, the relative weight of
the extra-regional networks has decreased since the end of the
Nineties. On the contrary, the share of U.S. originated compounds
that are licensed in the U.S. has risen from 61.2 percent in 1991-1997
to 65.70 percent in 1998-2004. Analogously, the share of EU-25 compounds licensed to local corporations has increased from 28.0 percent

Table IV.14   Licensing agreements (R&D and marketing), by nationality of the licensee and the licensor, 1991-2004

NATIONALITY OF THE LICENSOR		NATIONALITY OF THE LICENSEE					
1991-1997	Total	U.S.		EU-25		Other	
U.S.	1,588	971	61.15%	344	21.66%	273	17.19%
	70.36%	72.03%		67.19%		68.77%	
EU-25	410	225	54.88%	115	28.05%	70	17.07%
	18.17%	16.69%		22.46%		17.63%	
Other	259	152	58.69%	53	20.46%	54	20.85%
	11.48%	11.28%		10.35%		13.60%	
Total	2,257	1348	59.73%	512	22.68%	397	17.59%
1998-2004							
U.S.	2,321	1,525	65.70%	474	20.42%	322	13.87%
	65.79%	72.52%		54.05%		58.76%	
EU-25	769	347	45.12%	297	38.62%	125	16.25%
	21.80%	16.50%		33.87%		22.81%	
Other	438	231	52.74%	106	24.20%	101	23.06%
	12.41%	10.98%		12.09%		18.43%	
Total	3,528	2,103	59.61%	877	24.86%	548	15.53%

Source: our computations on Databiotech.com

Reading key: number of licensing agreements | as % of licensor's deals (total by row)
                   as % of licensee's deals (total by column) |

to 38.6 percent. Meanwhile, EU-25 originated compounds licensed to U.S. companies have decreased from 54.9 percent to 45.1 percent.

The share of out-licensing agreements by U.S. companies has decreased from 70.4 percent in 1991-1997 to 65.8 percent in 1998-2004, whereas no significant variation is registered in the share of in-licensing agreements. On the other side, EU-25 companies have increased their share of out-licensing agreements from 18.2 percent to 21.8 percent. Even the share of in-licensing agreement is increased (from 22.5 to 33.9 percent) to detriment of the share of U.S. inventions licensed to EU companies (from 67.2 to 54 percent).

This pattern shows that U.S. companies still play a predominant role in the network of licensing agreements, being present both as licensor and licensee in more than respectively 65 and 59 percent of the deals. In this respect, it is interesting to compare the information about the flow of products (analyzed in Chapter III) with the informa-

Table IV.15   Stage at signing of licensing agreements, by nationality of the licensee, 1991-2004

Stage at signing	U.S. & Canada			Europe			Japan			Others		
	no.	%	Cum %	no.	%	Cum %	no.	%	Cum %	no.	%	Cum %
From start	77	5.3	5.3	50	3.6	3.6	8	1.5	1.5	8	2.0	2.0
Preclinical	594	41.0	46.3	370	26.4	30.0	122	23.4	25.0	59	14.6	16.6
Clinical I	166	11.4	**57.7**	134	9.6	39.5	46	8.8	33.8	17	4.2	20.8
Clinical II	183	12.6	70.3	178	12.7	**52.2**	76	14.6	48.4	59	14.6	35.5
Clinical III	116	8.0	78.3	172	12.3	64.5	74	14.2	**62.6**	51	12.7	48.1
PreReg.	59	4.1	82.4	100	7.1	71.6	47	9.0	71.6	35	8.7	**56.8**
Registration	11	0.8	83.2	12	0.9	72.5	8	1.5	73.1	11	2.7	59.6
Market	244	16.8	100	386	27.5	100	140	26.9	100	163	40.4	100

Note: in bold the median stage at signing

Source: our computations on Databiotech.com

tion about the flow of technology as described by the R&D and marketing licensing agreements reported in Table IV.14. The analysis in Chapter III reported a negative trade balance for pharmaceutical products of the U.S. industry, while a positive "trade balance" of licensing agreements for the U.S. and a negative trade balance for the EU-25 countries emerge. Indeed, U.S. corporations licensed out 2,321 and licensed in 2,103 agreements in the period 1998-2004 (with a positive balance of 218 agreements), whereas EU-25 corporations registered a negative licensing balance equal to 108 agreements (877 agreements as licensee, and 769 agreements as licensor). In other words, the U.S. is a net exporter of intellectual property rights while the EU-25 has a trade deficit as far as innovative drugs are concerned. This further supports the hypothesis that the U.S. foreign direct investments in Europe are of "vertical resource seeking" type, whereas European investments in the U.S. are both horizontal "market seeking" and vertical "knowledge seeking" investment in R&D.

Table IV.15 reports the stage of the licensing agreements at signing. The majority of U.S. companies signs in license agreements in the early clinical phase or before, at a stage when they can still claim a high portion of value added from final drug sales. On the contrary, companies outside North America sign deals only at later stages, with a high proportion of them entering only at the commercialization stage (around 27 percent in Europe and Japan, 40 percent in other countries, whereas only 17 percent in North America). Indeed, more than 50 percent of the agreements are signing at Clinical I or before in the U.S. (with 46.3 percent being signed during preclinical or early discovery stages), at Clinical II or before in Europe, and at Clinical III or before in Japan. Corporations from other countries sign the largest part of the agreements they are involved in at the pre-registration stage or later.

Our results provide support to the claim that U.S. institutions play a prominent role in networks of innovative activities. The U.S. pioneered the rise of a new organization model of R&D activities in the pharmaceutical industry. It was based on an effective division of labor between smaller and larger companies with different comparative advantages in the exploration and exploitation of new innovative opportunities (March, 1991), whereas Europe has been less effective in encouraging the growth of new technology suppliers and innovation specialists. This fact has been emphasized by the increasing reliance of European drug multinationals on sources of research capabilities and innovation located in the U.S. thereby reinforcing the difficulties in creating a European industry of technological suppliers.

IV.5   National Systems of Innovation in Biopharmaceuticals

Since the U.S. and Europe constitute the main regional systems of innovation in pharmaceuticals, it is worth comparing their architectures in order to understand the role that different organizations play within them as well as the structure and dynamics of networks and markets for technologies. In this section, the focus is on the innovative activities and arrangements thereof, therefore we only consider collaborative R&D projects.[18]

Table IV.17 shows the number and percentage of collaborative agreements signed by Public Research Organizations ("PROs"), Dedicated Biotechnology Firms ("DBFs") and Established Companies ("ECs") in North America, Europe, and the rest of the world, as well as the change in these figures between 1991 and 2004.

PROs are public and private universities and hospitals involved in the pharmaceutical R&D. DBFs are high tech specialized start-up

---

[18] Marketing agreements are not considered in the analysis.

Table IV.16 Number of collaborative R&D Projects, by region and type of institution: 1991-1997 and 1998-2004

	projects originated								projects developed							
	total		PRO		DBF		EC		total		PRO		DBF		EC	
Regions	no.	%	no.	%	no.	%	no.	%	no.	%	no.	%	no.	%	no.	%
1991-1997																
U.S.	840	77.2	242	28.8	495	58.9	103	12.3	691	63.5	4	0.6	374	54.1	313	45.3
EU-25	165	15.2	54	32.7	72	43.6	39	23.6	206	18.9	0	0.0	63	30.6	143	69.4
Others	83	7.6	41	49.4	25	30.1	17	20.5	191	17.6	1	0.5	46	24.1	144	75.4
Total	*1088*	*100*	*337*	*31.0*	*592*	*54.4*	*159*	*14.6*	*1088*	*100*	*5*	*0.5*	*483*	*44.4*	*600*	*55.1*
1998-2004																
U.S.	940	66.4	218	23.2	638	67.9	84	8.9	878	62.0	8	0.9	561	63.9	309	35.2
EU-25	305	21.5	65	21.3	191	62.6	49	16.1	312	22.0	3	1.0	134	42.9	175	56.1
Others	171	12.1	49	28.7	96	56.1	26	15.2	226	16.0	4	1.8	110	48.7	112	49.6
Total	*1416*	*100*	*332*	*23.4*	*925*	*65.3*	*159*	*11.2*	*1416*	*100*	*15*	*1.1*	*805*	*56.9*	*596*	*42.1*

PRO = Public Research Organizations, DBF = Dedicated Biotech Companies, EC = Established Companies, mostly pharmaceutical companies.

Source: our computations on Databiotech.com

companies, while ECs are large pharmaceutical firms that, together with the production of pharmaceuticals for the market, also conduct intense R&D activities to improve their products and continuously find new pharmaceutical solutions.

DBFs play a central role in the U.S. innovation system, which have no analogue abroad, both as initiators and developers of new R&D projects. Their importance increased during the 1990s, to the extent that DBFs, complemented by PROs, currently initiate the largest share of collaborative R&D projects in the U.S. DBFs have also grown significantly in Europe since the early 1990s, but there are two marked differences with the U.S. First, the share of projects initiated and developed by DBFs is greater in the U.S. than in the EU-25. Second, North American DBFs differ from their European counterparts in being more frequently involved in later phases of development and commercialization of compounds.

DBFs play a crucial role in bridging the gap between the exploration of new research opportunities and market development of innovations generated outwardly.

Therefore, along all the observed years, specialization and division of innovative labor have been increasing in the U.S. system. On the one hand, PROs and DBFs have specialized in scanning the technological frontier in search of new therapeutic and technological opportunities. On the other hand, ECs have been maturing, selecting capabilities and increasingly specializing in downstream development of research opportunities originated elsewhere. Over time, a dense network of R&D collaborative agreements has been growing around the U.S. biotechnology industry to include all the most important pharmaceutical companies in the U.S., Europe and Japan. Most of them also decided to set up R&D laboratories in the U.S. biotech regions.

As long as division of labor increases and networks spread out, both American and (to a lower extent) European ECs lose important shares in the number of total projects they originated and developed. The share of projects developed by ECs over the total number of developed R&D projects has declined from 69.4 percent over the period 1991-1997 to 56.1 percent in 1998-2004. However, despite their diminished importance, ECs still play a pre-eminent role in the clinical development phase of compounds in most EU countries. The share of R&D projects developed by ECs over the period 1980-2004 for selected European countries (namely Italy, Spain, Netherlands, and Ireland) is about 80 percent or above.

Indeed, among European countries, only the UK, Belgium and Denmark resemble the U.S. model, while all other national innovation systems are largely different. Pharmaceutical innovation systems throughout Continental Europe remain predominantly centered around large pharmaceutical corporations, while North American DBFs play a crucial role in the international system of division of innovative labor. Hence, the European pharmaceutical systems of division of innovative labor are locked in an evolutionary phase antecedent to the one reached by the U.S. system. As a result, three DBFs have been able to stay independent and to enter the group of top forty wholly integrated pharmaceutical companies. All of them (Amgen, Genzyme and Biogen-Idec) are U.S.-based.[19]

---

[19] Two more are controlled by Swiss MNCs: Genentech by Hoffman-la-Roche and Chiron by Novartis.

Structural differences between the U.S. and Europe have also relevant implications in terms of the research areas targeted within each country. A different set of incentives is placed on firms, distinguishing small biotechnology enterprises from large pharmaceutical corporations, as compared to public research organizations, which respond differently to scientific and market-based incentives. For a long while, the theoretical literature has debated about the crucial factors driving firms' innovative research efforts, distinguishing them in "technology push" versus "demand pull" determinants, the former considering the exogenous effect of science on technological change, while the latter regard market growth and size as the only determinants of the decision to invest in R&D. Both views tell only a part of the story. The decision to invest in R&D, and therefore the rate and direction of technological progress, is the result of the interplay between the advances spanning from basic science, institutional variables, and economic factors, namely market growth and size (Dosi, 1982, 1988). Despite the fervor of the theoretical debate, little empirical evidence is provided on the role of demand and science in affecting the rate of technological progress.

In order to investigate the effect of market size and risk of failure on the entry of new drugs into a market and on pharmaceutical innovation, it is worthwhile to focus on two specific research areas—"orphan" diseases without therapy and African diseases—both characterized by a small market potential and high risk of failure (see also Appendix V.2). Following Schmookler's famous argument that "the amount of invention is governed by the extent of the market," Acemoglu and Linn (2004) have recently found a strong effect of the market size on the entry of non-generic drugs and new molecular entities. However, Arora *et al.* (2000) have argued that DBFs take full advantage of the Orphan Disease Act[20] and tend to focus on smaller markets in order to avoid potential competition with established pharmaceutical companies (see also Lerner, 1995). Indeed, biotechnology companies have undertaken the bulk of research in this area. As of 2000, biotechnology companies had sponsored 70 percent or more than 900 orphan-designated projects

---

[20] The U.S. Orphan Drug Act, which went into effect in 1983, created a number of financial incentives for biopharmaceutical companies to develop new drugs for diseases having a limited market. The primary attraction for companies under this legislation was a promise of seven years of market exclusivity, unless a follow-on product was approved that was deemed to be "clinically superior," i.e. characterized by a higher effectiveness or a better safety profile on a clinically meaningful endpoint.

Table IV.17   Number of R&D projects addressing diseases without therapy (DNET), by region and institution type of originators and developers (1980-2004)

	projects originated								projects developed							
	Total		PRO		DBF		EC		Total		PRO		DBF		EC	
	no.[1]	%	no.	%	no.	%	no.	%	no.	%	no.	%	no.	%	no.	%
U.S.	860	53.9	177	70.5	524	70.2	159	26.5	771	48.3	104	68.0	481	67.4	186	25.5
	100.0	+0.8	20.6	+1.0	60.9	+0.8	18.5	-0.4	100.0	+0.3	13.5	+0.9	62.4	+0.4	24.1	-0.8
EU-25	334	20.9	25	10.0	115	15.4	194	32.4	356	22.3	13	8.5	121	16.9	222	30.5
	100.0	-2.0	7.5	-3.0	34.4	-3.0	58.1	-0.9	100.0	-1.8	3.7	-3.2	34.0	-2.4	62.4	-1.2
Japan	138	8.6	15	6.0	2	0.3	121	20.2	169	10.6	12	7.8	2	0.3	155	21.3
	100.0	-0.5	10.9	+0.9	1.4	+0.6	87.7	+0.3	100.0	+0.5	7.1	+1.8	1.2	+1.6	91.7	+0.9
Other	264	16.5	34	13.5	105	14.1	125	20.9	300	18.8	24	15.7	110	15.4	166	22.8
	100.0	+2.1	12.9	-1.0	39.8	+2.4	47.3	+3.1	100.0	+2.5	8.0	-0.4	36.7	+2.5	55.3	+3.4
Total	1,596	100.0	251	100.0	746	100.0	599	100.0	1,596	100.0	153	100.0	714	100.0	729	100.0
	100.0	—	15.7	—	46.7	—	37.5	—	100.0	—	9.6	—	44.7	—	45.7	—

Table IV.18   Number of R&D projects on Africa's diseases (AD), by region and institution type of originators and developers (1980-2004)

	projects originated								projects developed							
	Total		PRO		DBF		EC		Total		PRO		DBF		EC	
	no.[1]	%	no.	%	no.	%	no.	%	no.	%	no.	%	no.	%	no.	%
U.S.	822	56.8	239	61.8	369	74.7	214	37.9	762	52.7	184	57.0	356	71.1	222	35.7
	100.0	+1.1	29.1	-0.0	44.9	+0.9	26.0	+1.7	100.0	+0.9	24.1	-0.5	46.7	+0.6	29.1	+1.1
EU-25	338	23.4	65	16.8	73	14.8	200	35.4	383	26.5	64	19.8	85	17.0	234	37.6
	100.0	-1.3	19.2	-0.5	21.6	-2.0	59.2	-0.4	100.0	-0.8	16.7	+0.8	22.2	-1.6	61.1	0.0
Japan	86	5.9	17	4.4	—	—	69	12.2	85	5.9	17	5.3	—	—	68	10.9
	100.0	-2.2	19.8	-1.9	—	-4.9	80.2	-2.0	100.0	-2.4	20.0	-1.6	—	-5.2	80.0	-2.1
Other	200	13.8	66	17.1	52	10.5	82	14.5	216	14.9	58	18.0	60	12.0	98	15.8
	100.0	+0.6	33.0	+1.4	26.0	-0.2	41.0	+0.4	100.0	+0.6	26.9	+1.4	27.8	+0.1	45.4	+0.4
Total	1446	100.0	387	100.0	494	100.0	565	100.0	1446	100.0	323	100.0	501	100.0	622	100.0
	100.0	—	26.8	—	34.2	—	39.1	—	100.0	—	22.3	—	34.6	—	43.0	—

Reading key and notes for both tables:

number of projects	as percent (%) of total by column
as percent (%) of total by row	as percent (%) with respect to Rest of the World[2]

PRO = Public Research Organizations, DBF = Dedicated Biotech Companies,
EC = Established Companies, mostly pharmaceutical companies.

Source: our computations on Databiotech.com

(1) All decimal numbers (0.0) are percentages (%). Non-decimal numbers are counts. (2) This figure is computed as the difference between relative effort within the country (number of projects in a given country targeting DNET as a percentage of the total number of R&D project in that country) and the relative effort in the Rest of the World. The figure is in bold if the difference is statistically different from zero at the 5 percent level.

in the U.S., and 50 percent of all approved biotechnology products had orphan drug status (Kettler and Marjanovic, 2004).

Table IV.18 considers R&D projects carried out from 1980 to 2002 and targeted to diseases for which no therapy exists, at least up to 2003.

More than 50 percent of R&D projects targeting diseases without therapy have been started by U.S. research organizations. Table IV.18 highlights the leading role of U.S. DBFs and PROs, which account for more than 70 percent of originated projects and of a high share of projects developed worldwide. DBFs play a prominent role within the field both as developer and as originator, even though a large share of projects worldwide is also developed by ECs, with important differences among the U.S. and the other regions considered in the analysis. While ECs developed 62.4 percent and 91.7 percent of the projects respectively developed within EU-25 and Japan, the figure drops to 24.1 percent in the U.S., where DBFs play the major role as developers (62.4 percent of U.S. developed projects).

A similar pattern emerges looking at the case of diseases affecting the Third World[21] or "African diseases" (see Table IV.18). Again, the leading role of the U.S. comes into evidence. U.S. institutions originated 56.8 percent of R&D projects targeted to African diseases and developed 52.7 percent. In this case both PROs and DBFs are involved. U.S. PROs originated 61.8 percent of R&D projects worldwide (and developed 57.0 percent), while U.S. DBFs originated 74.7 percent of worldwide projects targeted to African diseases, and developed 71.1 percent. Within the U.S., PROs account for approximately 29.1 percent of originated projects and 24.1 percent of the developed projects; while DBFs are responsible for approximately 44.9 percent of originated projects and 46.7 percent of the projects that have been developed. On the contrary, ECs play a prominent role in EU-25 and Japan.

The leading role of the U.S. in designing and developing R&D projects targeted to Africa's diseases and orphan diseases has some explanations. First, among the sets of orphan drug legislation that provide incentives for addressing R&D efforts on orphan drugs and neglected diseases, the U.S. Orphan Drug Act is the oldest one. It came into force in 1983, while orphan drug laws in Japan and in the EU have a more recent history (1993 and 2000 respectively). Second, the

---

[21] These have been selected on the basis of Cockburn and Janjouw (2001).

Orphan Drug Act has proven to be a strategy to develop the small biotech industry, which is the bulk of innovative activities carried out in the U.S. pharmaceuticals industry. In fact, many of the original biotech compounds were natural substances that were not eligible for patents. Given the uncertainty surrounding biotech patents, the exclusivity period guaranteed by the orphan drug legislations was an important market incentive to many biopharmaceutical firms. As a result, the U.S. Orphan Drug Act not only benefited existing DBFs, but also led to the establishment of a large number of new biotechnology firms as they were able to find a niche market in orphan drugs. Along with the introduction of incentives aimed at spurring the biotechnology industry, the U.S. Orphan Drug Act has been very successful in encouraging many new therapies for rare diseases that have provided significant health benefits to patients in terms of both quality of life and longevity in developed as well in developing countries (Lichtenberg and Waldfogel, 2003). It also acted to fill the existing lack of R&D investments in neglected diseases of poor countries. In this context, public interventions are needed to develop drugs targeted to orphan diseases, such as malaria and tuberculosis, given the insufficient revenues on the demand side and high fixed costs of R&D. However, the low ability of poor countries to pay for health care is such that there are too few investments carried out by developing economies. In addition, there has been a general reluctance of developed countries to come to their aid, at least until recently. In this sense, U.S. orphan drug legislation has provided an instructive model for other industrialized economies, especially for the EU, to act according to the public good nature of health care. In recent years, a number of public-private partnerships (PPPs) have emerged for the development of new vaccines and medicines targeting diseases widely spread in developing countries. Recently PPPs have altered the international framework in the pharmaceutical sector, as a new paradigm for drug development activities. They have resulted from a gradual convergence of private-for-profit operators and public sector (under pressure of international organizations such as the World Bank) leaning toward the exploration of new "open-source" organization models (Munos, 2006).

Another important aspect linked to the ability of the U.S. to operate in high-risk illness areas comes from the well-rooted presence of institutional investors. Venture capital organizations finance these high-risk, potentially high-reward projects, purchasing equity stakes while the firms are still privately held. Until recently, the venture capital industry was almost exclusively a U.S. centered phenomenon. Jeng and Wells (2000) estimated that in 1996 the U.S. venture capital pool was about three times larger than total venture capital pool in twenty-one other nations, of which 70 percent was in three countries with strong ties to the U.S.: Israel, Canada and the Netherlands. In the same paper Jeng and Wells find that not only is the strength of the initial public offering market of crucial importance for the commitment of venture capitalists, government policy can also have a dramatic impact on the venture capital industry. For instance, Kortum and Lerner (2000) focus on the surge of venture capital funds that occurred after 1978 in the U.S. when the Department of Labor freed pensions to invest in venture capital and find that venture funding does have a strong positive impact on innovation. According to their results a dollar of venture capital appears to be three to four times more potent in stimulating patenting than the same amount of traditional corporate R&D spending. Moreover, Hege *et al.* (2003) find out that U.S. venture capitalists outperform European ones in terms of internal rate of returns of the financed projects, concluding that either they are more sophisticated or they can benefit form network effects through "a web of institutions, experience and sufficiently transparent and deep markets and networks for human resources and knowledge". More recently, a movement called venture philanthropy has adopted techniques that worked well for venture capital firms in the 1990s to renew the U.S. philanthropic movement by affirming deeper interaction between giver and recipient and more emphasis on measurable outcomes. The importance of the biotechnology sector in the U.S. is sustained by the evolution of the U.S. stock market where the bio-pharmaceutical indices have constantly outperformed the Dow Jones I. A. and the S&P 500. In Europe the two indices have performed equally well, growing more than the D.J. Stoxx TMI. The similarity between the behavior in the two stock markets should not come as a surprise, given the globalized nature of the companies involved. Generally speaking, the stock market boom of the late 1990s greatly increased the favorable conditions for the flourishing of new biotech start-ups. However, while in Europe the bubble bursting caused a significant blow to biotech share prices, in the U.S. the situation was quite different. There, the fine grained R&D network and the highly competitive price structure constituted a breeding ground for the real beginning of new industrial sector, capable of continuing its activities well after the absorption of the high tech bubble. This sector is based on a fruitful and steady flow of collaborations between different kinds of R&D performers, accounting for a growing share of new drug development. Moreover, since biotech companies are a vital component of the R&D process, thanks to their light and flexible cost structure they also seize very large profit margins, and this contributes to explain their exceptional performances on the stock exchange. The profitable U.S. biopharmaceutical system of innovation cannot be easily replicated abroad, and this is the main reason why the difference between the U.S. and Europe is much more evident, when comparing quotations of biotech firms rather than of firms dealing with health care and pharmaceuticals more generally. Moreover, the U.S. biotechnology industry is sustained by institutional investors whose role in Europe is much more limited. In particular, the relevance of venture capital arises from some distinctive features of this sector. Information asymmetries and a great deal of uncertainty in biotechnology research make it difficult for contracting parties to define the feature of the product to be developed and to draft an enforceable agreement specifying the contributions of the R&D firms. In this context, venture capital helps biotech firms to finance R&D projects that otherwise would have been less likely to be funded through contract research with established pharmaceutical firms (Lerner *et al.*, 2003).

All in all, we can conclude that even if it is generally true that innovation is at least partially pulled by the potential market size, small biotechnology companies show a higher propensity to operate in risky and small markets—for instance orphan and neglected therapeutic areas. Hence, the rise of the biotech sector has generated large social returns. The support of a venture capital industry (and ultimately the stock market) has been essential. As Cockburn (2004) points out, "at least in the U.S. equity market, tolerance for risks has risen, and after well-hyped early successes, investors became comfortable with the idea of "high science for profit," developed a shared language and conceptual framework for valuing these new ventures, and—periodically—have been willing to support the new sector with substantial injections of capital."

Huge public R&D expenditures in the U.S. are complemented by dynamic financial institutions which help the U.S. private sector to

Figure IV.4 Stock market indices: global vs. health, pharmaceutical and biotechnology indices

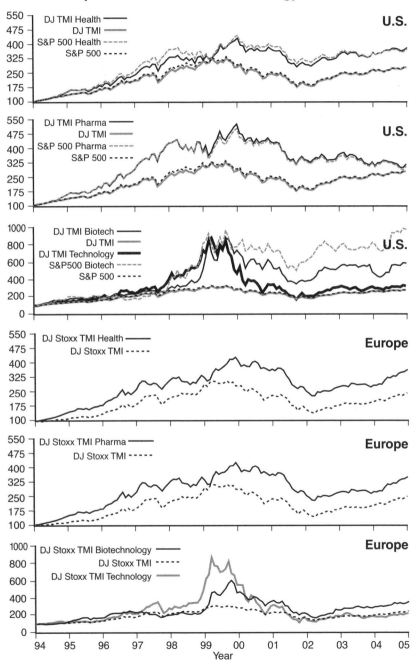

Source: www.bloomberg.com and www.stoxx.com

sustain the level of investment needed to research, develop and diffuse General Purpose Technologies able to increase pharmaceutical productivity in the long run.

Table A. IV.1 Licensing agreements by nationality of licensor and licensee: country breakdown, 1991-2004[1]

	(a)		Nationality of licensee						(b)		nationality of licensor						(a)-(b)	
	PROJECTS ORIGINATED		U.S.		EU-25		Other		PROJECTS DEVELOPED		U.S.		EU-25		Other			
Country	no.	%	no.	%	no.	%	no.	%	no.	%	no.	%	no.	%	no.	%	no.	%
U.S.	3909	67.57	2496	63.85	818	20.93	595	15.22	3451	59.65	2496	72.33	572	16.57	383	11.10	458	7.92
UK	491	8.49	222	45.21	181	36.86	88	17.92	570	9.85	326	57.19	186	32.63	58	10.18	-79	-1.37
Japan	159	2.75	91	57.23	38	23.90	30	18.87	343	5.93	237	69.10	67	19.53	39	11.37	-184	-3.18
Germany	226	3.91	103	45.58	89	39.38	34	15.04	327	5.65	186	56.88	106	32.42	35	10.70	-101	-1.75
Canada	258	4.46	124	48.06	61	23.64	73	28.29	188	3.25	95	50.53	38	20.21	55	29.26	70	1.21
France	147	2.54	72	48.98	48	32.65	27	18.37	172	2.97	98	56.98	45	26.16	29	16.86	-25	-0.43
Denmark	74	1.28	31	41.89	30	40.54	13	17.57	66	1.14	37	56.06	19	28.79	10	15.15	8	0.14
Italy	28	0.48	14	50.00	10	35.71	4	14.29	39	0.67	29	74.36	7	17.95	3	7.69	-11	-0.19
Belgium	37	0.64	21	56.76	11	29.73	5	13.51	46	0.80	26	56.52	14	30.43	6	13.04	-9	-0.16
Spain	13	0.22	11	84.62	2	15.38	0	0.00	25	0.43	15	60.00	6	24.00	4	16.00	-12	-0.21
Netherlands	40	0.69	20	50.00	16	40.00	4	10.00	45	0.78	28	62.22	13	28.89	4	8.89	-5	-0.09
Ireland	60	1.04	44	73.33	8	13.33	8	13.33	59	1.02	44	74.58	9	15.25	6	10.17	1	0.02
Sweden	41	0.71	21	51.22	15	36.59	5	12.20	28	0.48	19	67.86	6	21.43	3	10.71	13	0.22
Finland	13	0.22	7	53.85	1	7.69	5	38.46	3	0.05	3	100.00	0	0.00	0	0.00	10	0.17
Other EU-25	9	0.16	6	66.67	1	11.11	2	22.22	9	0.16	7	77.78	1	11.11	1	11.11	0	0.00
Switzerland	124	2.14	78	62.90	23	18.55	23	18.55	288	4.98	193	67.01	60	20.83	35	12.15	-164	-2.83
Norway	5	0.09	1	20.00	2	40.00	2	40.00	4	0.07	0	0.00	2	50.00	2	50.00	1	0.02
Other	151	2.61	89	58.94	35	23.18	27	17.88	122	2.11	70	57.38	28	22.95	24	19.67	29	0.50
Total	5785	100	3451	59.65	1389	24.01	945	16.34	5785	100	3909	67.57	1179	20.38	697	12.05	0	0.00

(1) In columns (a), (b) and (a)-(b) the percentages are based on the total number of projects. In the remaining columns the percentages are relative to the total number of projects originated or developed by country (totals by rows)

Source: our computations on Databiotech.com

Table A.IV.2   Number of collaborative R&D projects, by region and institution type of originators and developers: country breakdown, 1991-2004[1]

Country	(a) PROJECTS DEVELOPED no.	%	Developer PRO no.	%	DBF no.	%	EC no.	%	(b) PROJECTS ORIGINATED no.	%	Originator PRO no.	%	DBF no.	%	EC no.	%	(a)-(b) no.	%
U.S.	1780	71.09	460	25.80	1133	63.70	187	10.50	1569	62.66	12	0.80	935	59.60	622	39.60	211	8.43
UK	201	8.03	65	32.30	108	53.70	28	13.90	225	8.99	3	1.30	110	48.90	112	49.80	-24	-0.96
Japan	44	1.76	2	4.50	13	29.50	29	65.90	150	5.99	1	0.70	21	14.00	128	85.30	-106	-4.23
Switzerland	21	0.84	2	9.50	5	23.80	14	66.70	132	5.27	1	0.80	20	15.20	111	84.10	-111	-4.43
Germany	92	3.67	11	12.00	65	70.70	16	17.40	125	4.99	0	0.00	33	26.40	92	73.60	-33	-1.32
Canada	114	4.55	49	43.00	65	57.00	0	0.00	82	3.27	1	1.20	76	92.70	5	6.10	32	1.28
France	58	2.32	14	24.10	31	53.40	13	22.40	65	2.60	0	0.00	17	26.20	48	73.80	-7	-0.28
Denmark	25	1.00	1	4.00	13	52.00	11	44.00	22	0.88	0	0.00	10	45.50	12	54.50	3	0.12
Italy	9	0.36	5	55.60	2	22.20	2	22.20	14	0.56	0	0.00	2	14.30	12	85.70	-5	-0.20
Belgium	11	0.44	2	18.20	9	81.80	0	0.00	12	0.48	0	0.00	8	66.70	4	33.30	-1	-0.04
Spain	5	0.20	4	80.00	1	20.00	0	0.00	5	0.20	0	0.00	1	20.00	4	80.00	0	0.00
Netherlands	20	0.80	7	35.00	12	60.00	1	5.00	19	0.76	0	0.00	4	21.10	15	78.90	1	0.04
Ireland	18	0.72	1	5.60	0	0.00	17	94.40	18	0.72	0	0.00	0	0.00	18	100.00	0	0.00
Sweden	22	0.88	3	13.60	19	86.40	0	0.00	10	0.40	0	0.00	9	90.00	1	10.00	12	0.48
Finland	3	0.12	1	33.30	2	66.70	0	0.00	0	0.00	0	0.00	0	0.00	0	0.00	3	0.12
Norway	1	0.04	1	100.00	0	0.00	0	0.00	1	0.04	0	0.00	1	100.00	0	0.00	0	0.00
Other EU25	5	0.20	4	80.00	1	20.00	0	0.00	3	0.12	0	0.00	3	100.00	0	0.00	2	0.08
Other	75	3.00	37	49.30	38	50.70	0	0.00	52	2.08	2	3.80	38	73.10	12	23.10	23	0.92
Total	2504	100.00	669		1517		318		2504	100.00	20		1288		1196			

(1) Percentages are calculated on the total number of projects originated and developed in each country. PRO = Public Research Organizations, DBF = Dedicated Biotech Companies, EC = Established Companies, mostly pharmaceutical companies. Source: our computations on Databiotech.com.

Chapter V
Industry Structure and Competition

Chapter V

Industry Structure and Competition

Main Findings

- The U.S. market has experienced high growth rates over the period 1994-2004. Similar to most developed countries (including Japan and many EU countries), the rapid growth in the U.S. has been driven by the increase in drug consumption. However, the U.S. is the only case in which the growth in consumption has been paralleled by a sustained growth of drug prices.

- U.S. drug prices have been more than double the EU-15 average in the past decade. Branded drugs account for this gap, while the prices of U.S. generic drugs are tantamount to the EU-15 average. In Europe, less regulated markets such as the United Kingdom and Germany display higher prices than countries like France and Italy, which rely upon pervasive price regulation. U.S. prices of generic drugs are substantially aligned with the EU-15 average, but in many cases they are well below European and Canadian levels. More extensive prescribing and use of relatively less expensive generics in the United States has fostered a competitive generics market there, and has helped to free up financial resources that are used in turn to fund greater consumption of innovative drugs by patients for whom those medicines constitute the most appropriate and beneficial treatment option. By artificially constraining prices of innovative medicines while failing to stimulate a robust and competitive market for generic medicines, some European governments are missing the opportunity to create "headroom" for innovation.

- Generic penetration is much higher in the U.S., where generics account for 33.7 percent of sales in volume in 2004, compared to 16.3 percent in EU-15. In Italy and France the shares of generic drugs are lower than the EU average (5.1 percent and 11.3 percent of the market in 2004). In addition, price competition among generic producer is stronger in the U.S. than in Europe.

- It is difficult to make straightforward comparisons between pharmaceutical prices in the United States and Europe, due to the complexity of the market-based, decentralized, and competitive U.S. pricing environment. That complexity results from the decentralized and market-based mechanisms of price definition, as well as the wide range of public and private sector players involved in providing and purchasing health-related goods and services. Price comparisons using average wholesale prices of pharmaceuticals in the United States fail to reflect the rebates that pharmaceutical firms are frequently required to pay to large-scale purchasers (especially government agencies), as well as price reductions frequently granted to private firms in return for high-volume purchase commitments. As a consequence, we complement cross-country price comparisons with a focus on industry structure and dynamics within countries. Our analysis documents why and how the U.S. pricing and competitive system is a key ingredient of industrial competitiveness.

- The comparison of concentration indices at the level of therapeutic submarkets shows that the U.S. pharmaceutical market is more concentrated than the European one. However, the higher concentration of the U.S. market does not imply lower market competition. On the contrary, product and firm turnover in the U.S. market turn out to be higher by far than in Europe. On average, market leadership in the U.S. can be sustained for less than six years, while the average for Europe is higher than nine years. This phenomenon relates to the intensity of firm turnover, which in the U.S. is almost double the European average.

- The high concentration of U.S. markets is due to the "premium price" that leading products are able to charge: larger price premiums with respect to the market average are granted to new products in the U.S. (+44 percent) as compared to Europe (+22 percent) and Japan (+15 percent).

- The U.S. market has high product turnover: entry and exit rates are around 50 percent more than in EU-15 and Japan.

- Innovative drugs are launched first in the U.S. and then in other major European markets: with respect to the EU-15, the median launch is delayed of eight months (17 months in the case of EU-25).

- The U.S. market sustains higher price differentiation and promotes dynamic competition at both the product and the firm levels, through a price engine mechanism. Diffusion of new products is faster in the U.S. than in Europe, both for branded and generic products.

- Government intervention into the market, in particular through price ceilings and restriction of patent protection, reduces firm mobility and incentives to sustain sunk cost investments in R&D and capital accumulation. Thus, markets are more static (less competitive) and consumer welfare decreases since a higher share of the healthcare expenditures is allocated to older and/or less innovative drugs.

- Health care and pharmaceutical expenditures are becoming topical and sensitive issues in the U.S. politics. In an open economy, any potential reform of the U.S. model has to be seen as a challenge not only for the U.S., but for all industrialized countries as well. The same is true for the effect of welfare reforms in Europe.

V.1 Overview

In this chapter we investigate the relationship between industrial performance and certain distinctive features of national pharmaceutical markets, including industry structure, intensity of competition as measured by firm and product turnover, entry of new molecules, and generic products.

When taking the effects of market structure on innovative performance and incentives to R&D into account, we need to distinguish between static and dynamic efficiency and to analyze their trade-off (see Ahn, 2002).

On the one hand, a competitive environment facilitates efficient resource allocation and can spur the invention of new or improved products, services, or processes. The resulting innovation can boost national economic growth and living standards (see FTC, 2003). The pharmaceutical industry is particularly important in this respect, being the source of new and more effective drugs that have certainly contributed to increase prosperity and improve quality of life (Lichtenberg, 2003).

On the other hand, competition is not necessarily conducive to rapid technological change. In particular, firms will be incentivized to invest in R&D only if they can expect some form of transient ex post market power. In addition, market power also helps to reduce uncertainty associated with excessive rivalry and duplication of R&D efforts, uncertainty that tends to undermine the incentive to invest.

All in all, as highlighted by a report of the Federal Trade Commission, competition and patents (accruing to the holder transient monopoly power) can together foster innovation, but a proper balance among the two measures needs to be reached for them to be effective (FTC, 2003).

On the one hand, European governments have widely ruled the pharmaceutical systems with a wide variety of measures aimed at cost containment focusing both on limiting demand or regulating prices. As a result, Europe is characterized by quite different healthcare systems in terms of the extent of market regulation and price control. On the other hand, the U.S. government does not directly influence the prices and demand of pharmaceuticals and allows drug prices to be determined by market competition. GOP (2000) has shown that there is too little market-based competition in the final markets in some of the European countries that has contributed to nurture inefficient positions within the industry, with implied effects on firms' innovation and market performances.

Most of the analyses in this chapter rely upon IMS Health data, reporting drug sales in 28 countries, including the U.S., Canada, China, India, Japan, and the EU-25 countries (with the exclusion of Cyprus and Malta), over the period 1994-2004. For each drug package, the IMS Health database covers information on the international product name, molecule/s, the ATC classification, the manufacturer's name, launch date, quantities sold expressed in SU (standard units),[1] the total value of sales at manufacturer's price, and other useful information.

---

[1] Standard units are habitually employed as a rough proxy for a dose to measure quantities of pharmaceutical products and are defined as one tablet, one capsule or 5 milliliters of a liquid product.

In the first section, we analyze the causes of the unprecedented growth in pharmaceutical expenditures during the last fifteen years. In the second section, we deconstruct the market structure and dynamics by means of market share concentration, mobility indices, and product turnover. In the third one, we provide price comparisons at the molecule level for EU-15 and the U.S. Next, we focus on product launch, and life cycle. All in all, we analyze the effect of market regulation on competition and incentives to innovation, taking into account both static and dynamic efficiency. In the Appendix, we perform a simulation exercise showing how price cuts and reductions in patent term impinge on firm mobility and limit the competitive strategies adopted by companies. Episodes of highly positive (and negative) sales performances become more and more unlikely. Thus, markets are more static (less competitive) and consumer welfare decreases since a higher share of the healthcare expenditures is allocated to older and/or less innovative drugs.

V.2 The Determinants of Market Growth

During the last decade, the U.S. pharmaceutical industry has experienced impressive rates of domestic sales growth. To identify the determinants of the upsurge of drug spending in the United States *vis-à-vis* the rest of the world, we use price index formulae analogous to those used by the U.S. Bureau of Labor Statistics and in Berndt (2001, 2002) as well as in Danzon and Pauly (2002). Likewise, we provide an accounting decomposition of the growth in ex-factory sales into three components:

1. The price increases for existing products, i.e. the change in spending if last year's mix of drugs were purchased today;

2. The portion of the growth in spending attributable to the uptake of new drugs launched in each year;

3. The residual component of pharmaceutical market growth due to increases in consumption volume and shifts to more expensive incumbent products.

Pharmaceutical price comparisons between the United States and Europe are rarely straightforward, due mainly to the complexity of the pricing environment. That complexity results from the decentralized and market-based or administrative-based nature of pricing decisions,

Figure V.1   The U.S. pharmaceutical market: sales growth and its components (1995-2004)

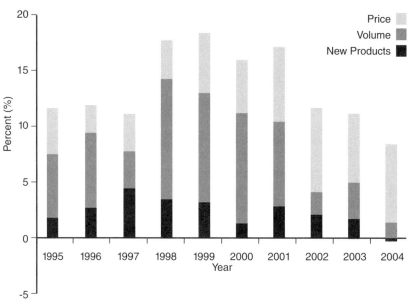

Source: our computations on IMS Health, Copyright 2005.

as well as the wide range of public- and private-sector players involved in providing and purchasing health-related goods and services. Average wholesale prices of pharmaceuticals in the United States and Europe fail to reflect the rebates that pharmaceutical firms are frequently required to pay to large-scale purchasers (especially government agencies), as well as price reductions frequently granted to private firms in return for high-volume purchase commitments.

As shown in Figure V.1, although expenditures on pharmaceuticals in the U.S. grew at roughly similar average annual rates of 11 percent between 1995 and 1997 and again after 2001, growth exceeded 16 percent per annum in the period 1998-2001. Until 1997, new drug launches had driven the growth of pharmaceutical expenditures followed by an increase in the utilization rate of drugs and broader coverage, while after 1997 the decline in new drug launches contributed to the decline in this element of market growth (see Chapter IV). In the last few years, the increase in drug prices has become the main component of total drug spending growth.

Figure V.2   U.S. prescription drug coverage by source of funds, historical data (1965-2005) and projections (2006-2015)[1]

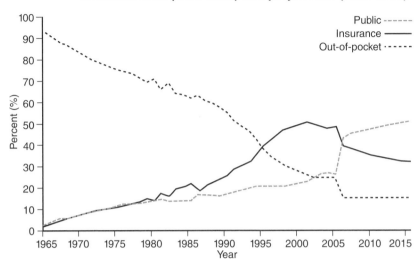

(1) The health spending projections were based on the 2004 version of the NHE released in January 2006.

Source: our computations on data from the Center for Medicare and Medicaid Services, Office of the Actuary for the U.S. National Health Expenditure Accounts.

In the second half of the 1990s, the growth in utilization and shifting to more expensive products, rather than price increases, has been the primary driver of the upsurge of pharmaceutical spending in most countries, including the United States. Although new products have surely contributed to the growth in utilization, the dramatic increase in drug spending is largely due to the drop in out-of-pocket payments and the moral hazard effects stemming from the growth of insurance coverage (see Figure V.2).

Indeed, the slowdown in drug spending in 2002-2004 is due both to contingent and persistent factors such as increased availability and consumption of generic drugs and more people covered under tiered co-payment drug plans (Heffler *et al.*, 2005).

In fact, U.S. prices of generic drugs are substantially aligned with the EU-15 average, and in many cases they are well below European and Canadian prices for generics. More extensive prescribing and use of relatively less expensive generics in the United States has fostered a competitive generics market, and has helped to free up financial resources that are used in turn to fund greater consumption of innovative drugs by patients for whom those medicines constitute the most appropriate and beneficial treatment option. By artificially constraining the prices of innovative medicines while failing to stimulate a robust and competitive market for generic medicines, European governments are missing the opportunity to create "headroom" for innovation.

However, moral hazard problems are expected to be amplified starting from January 2006 by the introduction of Medicare Part D which is likely to drive further reductions in out-of-pocket spending and a smaller decline in third-party pharmaceutical expenditure. McFadden (2006) estimates that moral hazard will increase the number of prescriptions and then the cost of the program by $6.8 billion. The creation of a market for multiple carriers and plans in the Part D legislation can only partially countervail the moral hazard problem as the reduction in out-of-pocket spending will primarily affect those Medicare beneficiaries who now lack drug coverage at all and those in Medigap plans that have high out-of-pocket payments. On the contrary, so far prescription drug price inflation seem not to have been influenced by Medicare Part D: Berndt *et al.* (2007) show that the pharmaceutical consumer price index was 4.25 percent annually form January 2000 to the passage of the initial legislation in June 2003, fell to about 3.7 percent before the implementation of Medicare Part D in January 2006, and since then has risen slightly to an AAGR of 4.06 percent.

The U.S. recorded a compound annual growth in 1994-2004 of 12.2 percentage points, among the top growth rates in the OECD countries. Like most developed countries including Japan and most EU countries, the growth in the U.S. has been driven by the increase in drug consumption, but the U.S. is the only case in which the growth in consumption has been paralleled by a sustained growth of drug prices.

Moreover, prices are the main driver of market growth in 2004. In this respect, it is worth noting the case of Germany and Italy as instances of regulation of prescriptions and drug prices respectively. The effects of the applied policies can be observed when analyzing the determinants of market growth in 2004.

Table V.1 The growth of pharmaceutical sales and its components: new products, price, volume and mix, 1994-2004

Country	Growth components	1994-2004 (%) [1]	2004 (%)
Japan	New products	1.00	0.61
	Price	-2.13	-3.07
	Volume & mix	5.17	6.92
	Total	*4.01*	*4.46*
France	New products	1.59	2.22
	Price	1.78	2.22
	Volume & mix	1.00	1.85
	Total	*4.38*	*6.29*
Germany	New products	1.69	1.99
	Price	2.28	1.69
	Volume & mix	1.96	-1.90
	Total	*5.96*	*1.78*
Italy	New products	1.33	1.70
	Price	2.27	-0.79
	Volume & mix	2.77	3.30
	Total	*6.34*	*4.22*
UK	New products	0.59	0.47
	Price	0.57	2.06
	Volume & mix	5.67	1.85
	Total	*6.83*	*4.37*
India	New products	3.27	3.66
	Price	2.83	0.68
	Volume & mix	0.66	2.28
	Total	*6.93*	*6.62*
Spain	New products	1.76	1.38
	Price	2.26	3.06
	Volume & mix	4.95	3.14
	Total	*8.99*	*7.58*
U.S.	New products	2.26	1.42
	Price	4.81	7.13
	Volume & mix	5.17	-0.47
	Total	*12.22*	*8.07*
China	New products	4.19	7.95
	Price	-4.81	-4.21
	Volume & mix	13.75	24.24
	Total	*13.09*	*27.98*

(1) Compound Annual Growth Rate (CAGR)

Source: our computations on IMS Health, Copyright 2005.

Table V.2   Inflation rate of pharmaceutical products vs. total manufacturing inflation rate[1]—in national currencies (NC) and U.S. dollars ($), 1995-2003, average

	inflation rate for pharmaceuticals in NC	inflation rate for pharmaceuticals in $ (A)	inflation rate for manufacturing in NC	inflation rate for manufacturing in $ (B)	A-B
France	-1.10	-1.61	-0.23	-0.74	-0.87
Germany	-0.76	-1.49	1.01	0.28	-1.77
Italy	0.60	-0.08	1.99	1.31	-1.39
UK	0.18	0.92	0.75	1.49	-0.57
U.S.	1.73	1.73	-0.83	-0.83	2.56

(1) Ex-factory production price indices (percentage values).

Source: our calculations on IMS Health, Copyright 2005; general inflation rate from OECD-STAN, 2004

In summer 2003, the Bundestag and Bundesrat passed the Statutory Health Insurance Modernization Act (SHIM Act), which came into force on January 1, 2004. The SHIM act was part of Chancellor Gerhard Schroeder's Agenda 2010, which aimed to make the German welfare state more internationally competitive by balancing solidarity with self-responsibility and making health care delivery more efficient. The reform discouraged physician consultations and prescribing by setting a new system of cost sharing consisting of a flat-rate user charge (€10) and additional co-payments for drug priced above the reference price. The flat-rate user charge has to be paid at least once quarterly on the first contact with a general practitioner (GP). Compared to 2003, visits to statutory health insurance (SHI) physicians subsequently dropped by 4.6 percent in the first quarter of 2004. As a result, the SHIM led to a fall-off in prescribing of -1.9 percent in volumes and Germany turned out to be one of the countries with the lowest growth rate for drug spending in 2004, and the only EU-15 country with a negative growth attributable to changes in volume and mix.

In Italy, a radical change in price dynamics was induced by Law number 202, August 2, 2004 which requires companies to apply a discount equivalent to a 6.8 percent ex-factory price reduction to their sales of reimbursable products to wholesalers and pharmacists. The Decree caused a sudden decrease of drug prices (-0.79 percent) partially offset by an increase of usage of both new and incumbent drugs. In particular, Italy has registered a +3.3 percent growth in the volume and mix component, the highest value among the largest European

The Fisher Chain Index

The Fisher index ("FI") is given by the simple geometric average of the correspondent Laspeyres ("LI") and Paasche ("PI") indices, where

the Laspeyres index is given by $LI = \dfrac{\Sigma p_i^t q_i^0}{\Sigma p_i^0 q_i^0}$

and the Paasche index by $PI = \dfrac{\Sigma p_i^t q_i^t}{\Sigma p_i^0 q_i^t}$.

where i indicates the sample of products sold both in period "0" and in period "t", p_i is the market price of the i-th product and q_i its quantity sold on the market (either in period "0" and in period "t").

By combining these two indices, the Fischer index aims at correcting the bias of each of them, due to the fact the former uses quantities in the first year to weight prices, while the latter uses quantities in the last year (of the period over which we want to measure inflation).

Taking a Fisher chain means to select, for each couple of continuous years, the sample of products marketed in both years, then measuring inflation with the Fisher index applied to that sample. The Fisher index is given by

$FI = \sqrt{(LI)(PI)}$.

The simple geometric average is preferred thanks to its properties. Linear and exponential transformations of all the elements considered in the average symmetrically apply to the average value.

countries included in the Table and higher than the average growth rate in the volume and mix component over the period 1994-2004 (equal to 2.77 percent).

The case of the UK is quite different. Most market growth in the period 1994-2004 came from volume and mix—the highest rate of growth for this element among the top EU-5 markets during this period. This reflects slow take up of new products, as shown in Figure V.4. Price increases are low as a succession of industry Government agreed five-year PPRS profit control schemes have combined pricing freedom at launch with subsequent price restrictions. Product introduction lags are low (see Figure V.5). The UK has a competitive unbranded generic market with high share by volume (31 percent—close to the U.S. figure of 33 percent, see Table A.V.1). The combined UK approach to competition and regulation stimulates R&D. The UK has the highest share of R&D as a percentage of pharmaceutical production of the EU-15 (see Table IV.2).

Table V.2 compares pharmaceutical price variations to the inflation rate of total manufacturing. The pharmaceutical price variation has been calculated using a Fisher chain index.[2] The U.S. average annual pharmaceutical inflation rate exceeds the economy-wide rate of inflation by almost three percent, while in the major European markets the pharmaceutical inflation rate is lower than that of total manufacturing. Berndt et al. (2007) reports that between January 1996 and October 2006 the BLS' Medical Consumer Price Index (MCPI) has raised about half again as fast as the overall CPI (these average annual growth rates were 3.86 percent and 2.50 percent, respectively).

The difference in the pharmaceutical relative price dynamics between the U.S. and the other European countries sum up approximately to 1.5 to three percentage points. As for future trends of pharmaceutical prices in the U.S., three issues have to be considered. First, the wave of patent expiry of blockbuster drugs and the increase of the market share of generics in the U.S. will contribute to reduce pharmaceutical inflation rates. Second, quality improvement and product innovation have to be distinguished from pure inflation, and higher

---

[2] The Fisher chain index measures price variations year by year taking into account only the products sold on the market in both years. The weight assigned to each product is changed every year in order to properly represent the product share in the basket of the quantities sold each year.

prices in the U.S. are related to a faster and wider diffusion of new and better drugs (U.S. Senate Finance Committee, 1996). Besides being a source of potential concern as for inflation, the U.S. price dynamic in pharmaceuticals is a factor of industrial competitiveness. To investigate further this statement, we need to analyze prices in the context of market competition, which is the object of the following sections.

V.3   Market Competition

The extent of market competition is captured by both market concentration and turnover (Vernon, 1971). While it has been widely recognized that concentration statistics provide only an imperfect measure of the intensity of competition, they are often used in competition policy, building on the argument that concentration and mobility are closely related. Concentrated industries are frequently described as having formidable barriers to both entry and internal mobility. We will show that this is not the case in pharmaceuticals. Moreover, concentration measured at the industry level can provide a misleading picture, since the pharmaceutical industry is composed of many therapeutic classes and of a wide range of technologies that when targeted to different diseases do not directly compete among each other (Sutton, 1998).

The simplest measure of market concentration is provided by the concentration ratio of the first n firms/products C_n (n = 1,...,10) in the market. Thus, the one-firm/product concentration ratio C_1 corresponds to the market share of the largest firm/product, while the C_n index equal the sum of the market shares of the top n firms/products in terms of sales. Thanks to data availability, the market concentration of the first product in nominal values can be decomposed into two parts: the concentration in real values—i.e. the number of standard units sold—multiplied by its relative price (the price of the first product divided by the mean price in the market).

Overall, the U.S. market is more concentrated than all the major EU markets (Germany, France, Italy and Spain, but not the UK), as well as Japan, China and India. On average, the three leading products in each of the top one hundred therapeutic categories account for 85.6 percent of total market share in the U.S., as compared with a total market share of 77.3 percent in the EU-25. It is clear that European markets are much more fragmented than the U.S. market. The U.S. market is as concentrated as the European one in terms of volume, while it is the most concentrated in terms of sales value. To a large extent, the high concentration of the U.S. market is due to the "premium price" that leading products can command. Indeed, the relative price of the market leader in the U.S. is 44 percent higher than the market average price—more than that in Europe (22 percent) or Japan (15 percent). We can conclude that the skewed nature of relative price distribution boosts the concentration level of the U.S. market.

Contrary to many other high-tech industries, the pharmaceutical industry remains fairly fragmented. In all countries, pharmaceutical industry concentration at the corporate level is lower than at the market level, since the pharmaceutical industry is composed of several independent submarkets (Sutton, 1998). Higher concentration in the U.S. market does not imply less competition. On the contrary, firm turnover in the U.S. is almost double that of the EU-15 and EU-25.

In fact, despite the premium price effect favoring the leading product, the U.S. market is far more competitive than European ones. Figure V.3 shows the product mobility index for each therapeutic market (ATC4 class) defined as the sum of the annual change in the product market share (Hymer and Pashigian, 1962). Boxplots in Figure V.2 highlight the median value of the index and the 75th and 25th percentiles of the distribution. Emergent markets are characterized by the highest level of market turnover, followed by Germany, the U.S., all other European markets and then Japan, which is characterized by the highest stability.

Not only the size of the market but also the nature of competition and regulation directly impinge on industrial competitiveness.

Market fragmentation undermines European companies by limiting the breadth of the market segment within which they can draw customers away from rivals, the most favorable outcome corresponding to the case where a new and improved product displaces all existing products within a given therapeutic market. As we have argued in Chapter III, even if the benefits of internal market size decrease with the extent of international integration of pharmaceutical markets thus leading to an increasing fragmentation of markets in Europe, centrifugal forces have to be counterbalanced by a process of market integra-

Table V.3 Average market concentration (sales and volumes) and relative prices of the first three products on the market, top 100 ATC4 classes, 1994-2004

	$C_1(S)$	$C_1(Q)$	P_1	$C_2(S)$	$C_2(Q)$	P_2	$C_3(S)$	$C_3(Q)$	P_3
EU-25	41.72	34.70	1.20	64.61	56.95	1.13	77.31	71.47	1.08
EU-15	41.18	34.17	1.21	63.83	56.05	1.14	76.53	70.49	1.09
Japan	39.77	34.61	1.15	62.74	54.75	1.15	78.25	69.36	1.13
U.S.	49.72	34.63	1.44	74.96	59.48	1.26	85.56	70.74	1.21
India	21.98	21.80	1.01	37.06	38.10	0.97	47.21	47.96	0.98
Germany	29.97	22.94	1.31	47.42	38.49	1.23	58.87	50.95	1.16
China	36.15	19.20	1.88	56.78	32.31	1.76	67.62	39.95	1.69
Italy	36.68	33.49	1.10	57.57	54.07	1.06	71.49	67.14	1.06
France	39.01	31.21	1.25	64.88	54.45	1.19	78.18	71.16	1.10
Spain	40.36	32.62	1.24	62.37	52.72	1.18	75.94	67.92	1.12
Canada	42.03	32.68	1.29	65.71	54.51	1.21	79.35	69.12	1.15
Latvia	45.07	35.23	1.28	68.63	63.24	1.09	82.96	79.67	1.04
Czech Rep.	46.26	40.80	1.13	72.70	66.68	1.09	86.77	83.83	1.04
Portugal	46.73	39.65	1.18	70.41	61.34	1.15	84.32	79.63	1.06
Belgium	48.33	42.24	1.14	76.64	70.27	1.09	92.24	86.65	1.06
Austria	48.43	41.12	1.18	74.19	66.51	1.12	87.70	82.03	1.07
Netherlands	48.56	37.60	1.29	72.35	58.42	1.24	86.24	76.38	1.13
Luxemburg	49.54	39.93	1.24	76.49	68.20	1.12	89.91	83.20	1.08
Slovak Rep.	50.02	42.52	1.18	76.77	72.70	1.06	90.69	90.27	1.00
Poland	50.16	39.71	1.26	76.55	68.63	1.12	89.29	85.30	1.05
Ireland	51.19	43.77	1.17	77.50	72.42	1.07	91.76	87.10	1.05
Lithuania	51.53	44.06	1.17	77.37	72.95	1.06	90.67	88.95	1.02
Finland	52.30	45.58	1.15	78.95	73.26	1.08	92.65	89.54	1.03
Greece	52.73	43.08	1.22	78.00	69.76	1.12	88.90	83.08	1.07
Denmark	53.50	45.22	1.18	80.34	75.33	1.07	93.07	91.05	1.02
Sweden	53.68	44.70	1.20	79.70	75.51	1.06	91.60	89.95	1.02
Estonia	54.71	45.13	1.21	80.74	75.51	1.07	93.32	91.67	1.02
Hungary	54.85	52.29	1.05	84.04	82.19	1.02	96.11	95.72	1.00
UK	55.69	48.34	1.15	79.61	75.16	1.06	90.20	87.75	1.03
Slovenia	61.25	54.13	1.13	88.25	84.98	1.04	97.89	97.47	1.00

Source: our computations on IMS Health, Copyright 2005.

Figure V.3   Product mobility statistics over all ATC4 therapeutic markets*

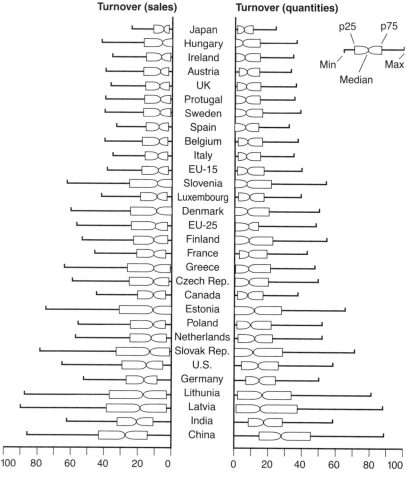

*The product mobility index is computed as in Hymer, Pashigian (1962), outliers have been omitted.
Source: our computations on IMS Health, Copyright 2005.

tion at the EU level, in order to improve competition in EU pharmaceutical markets.

The lower turnover of EU markets translates into a higher persistency and a lower contestability of the leading products. The U.S.

Table V.4 Market shares of the leading company (C₁) and top three companies (C₃) and firm turnover, sales and volumes, 2004

Country	C_1 Sales	C_1 Quantity	C_3 Sales	C_3 Quantity	Turnover* Sales	Turnover* Quantity
EU-15	9.59	8.43	25.00	21.11	5.77	5.23
EU-25	9.40	8.29	24.78	21.24	5.76	5.04
U.S.	15.14	9.33	31.06	20.12	9.48	10.55
Japan	6.59	13.59	17.47	23.43	5.49	4.52
Italy	10.20	7.33	23.85	19.22	5.46	4.91
Belgium	12.31	8.02	29.14	21.16	5.71	5.42
Spain	9.84	6.34	21.96	16.70	6.17	5.24
France	16.95	14.77	30.92	29.94	6.22	5.69
Portugal	8.43	7.80	23.93	19.10	6.83	5.32
Germany	7.60	12.20	19.88	26.77	7.23	6.92
Finland	11.79	23.94	31.14	38.60	7.25	4.91
Ireland	14.88	15.61	33.45	30.95	7.41	6.45
Luxembourg	12.35	7.17	32.03	21.16	7.56	6.07
Austria	7.95	10.18	23.03	23.74	7.80	5.74
Greece	10.63	13.49	28.00	29.06	8.34	8.31
Canada	15.02	13.45	28.96	29.47	8.70	12.43
Sweden	14.52	21.87	32.96	43.88	8.84	7.16
UK	15.72	19.56	35.73	35.83	9.16	5.22
Hungary	9.86	19.34	28.96	38.38	9.84	7.68
Netherlands	10.72	15.55	27.37	33.42	10.05	8.70
Denmark	9.96	34.72	26.48	55.36	10.23	17.86
Slovenia	17.93	21.10	40.54	47.41	10.96	9.53
Poland	7.62	12.33	21.72	29.59	11.42	8.97
India	6.50	9.89	16.64	22.53	11.68	11.59
Czech Rep.	14.30	26.03	27.64	36.79	12.26	9.56
Estonia	9.33	7.04	24.36	19.36	13.94	16.72
Slovak Rep.	10.97	22.44	25.83	38.70	14.78	11.68
Lithuania	7.73	7.00	21.60	18.35	21.23	19.05
Latvia	7.58	6.20	19.39	16.83	21.98	22.89
China	2.80	5.71	6.62	9.81	26.43	25.51

*computed as in Hymer, Pashigian, 1962.

Source: our computations on IMS Health, Copyright 2005.

average expected persistency of the leading product is slightly less than 6 years, while in the EU it is almost 10 years and in Japan more than 15 years (see Table V.5).

As shown in Table V.6, the U.S. market has the highest product turnover. The U.S. rate is 50.9 percent higher than the EU-15, and 49.9 percent higher than Japan. The most striking difference is found in product exit rate, which is on average 85.9 percent higher in the U.S. than in the EU-15, and 40.7 percent higher than in Japan. Product entry rates are 36.4 percent higher in the U.S. than in the EU-15, and 39.6 percent higher than in Japan. Therefore, the process of creative destruction is much more intense in the U.S. market than in European or Japanese markets.

However, within Europe a large variety of market and administrative settings coexists. In previous chapters we have identified two groups of countries: on one side, the northern European countries, characterized by high labor productivity, capital intensity and value added growth rates (cf. Chapter II), whose companies are the most internationalized (cf. Chapter III); on the other side, the EU continental and Mediterranean countries with firms mainly specialized in low-price pharmaceuticals and with low outward openness. These countries are also less exposed to foreign direct investment and are less competitive in terms of R&D (cf. Chapter IV). Data in Table V.7 confirm this view. Indeed, southern EU countries are characterized by high shares of local non-multinational companies.[3]

The strong presence of small less competitive and less productive local firms is due, at least partially, to tight price regulation systems. Indeed, on one hand they reduce the returns to investment in R&D, thus determining a sort of "adverse selection" which discriminates against the more innovative companies. On the other hand, strong regulatory policies coupled with international reference price scheme (such as the European mean price) can prevent multinational companies to enter low price markets so to avoid generalized price reductions (cfr. Appendix V). Final market regulation can thus distort private investment decisions.

Finally, the U.S. market is characterized by the greatest amount of competition in the off-patent segment of the market. On the one side,

---

[3] The high value of the market share hold by local firms in Japan is probably due to the low outward openness traditionally characterizing this country (cf. Cap III).

Table V.5 The persistence of the leading product in top 100 ATC4 markets

Country	Leadership change (%)										AP
	1995	1996	1997	1998	1999	2000	2001	2002	2003	2004	
Japan	7.22	4.12	6.65	4.85	4.29	10.58	7.52	8.00	6.77	6.03	15.15
Portugal	6.42	6.36	7.62	9.26	7.74	4.95	5.86	9.88	8.72	9.06	13.18
Spain	6.50	9.97	7.20	10.37	7.33	9.74	7.95	6.98	8.55	8.53	12.03
Italy	7.40	9.72	8.14	9.14	7.79	7.01	9.84	7.51	9.66	7.41	11.96
Sweden	4.99	10.69	9.62	7.93	10.56	8.62	7.43	10.70	9.30	8.66	11.30
UK	10.46	8.92	8.00	8.71	10.16	8.38	9.11	9.50	8.16	7.24	11.28
Ireland	11.39	10.00	11.39	9.17	9.01	6.61	8.16	10.91	11.82	7.42	10.43
Belgium	8.36	7.24	7.56	9.58	9.78	11.36	9.86	10.31	11.52	11.08	10.35
Finland	7.76	9.67	9.85	9.79	10.88	9.50	7.19	11.24	11.31	12.06	10.08
Austria	7.32	9.38	10.09	11.31	8.92	10.54	13.84	9.53	11.78	9.82	9.75
EU-15	10.70	10.94	9.84	10.71	10.15	9.34	10.23	10.25	10.81	10.16	9.70
EU-25	10.95	11.14	10.05	10.97	10.43	9.52	10.30	10.36	10.89	10.40	9.52
France	9.30	10.57	9.82	12.01	10.42	10.28	10.00	11.00	12.76	11.28	9.31
Luxembourg	12.30	10.71	13.44	11.08	11.05	9.89	8.11	10.33	10.11	10.63	9.29
Hungary	14.46	14.98	13.67	12.67	10.67	9.86	5.26	9.73	7.07	10.93	9.15
Netherlands	9.61	10.59	11.54	10.18	14.24	10.85	11.08	10.39	9.04	12.28	9.11
Denmark	12.33	13.38	11.18	12.54	13.61	9.81	8.97	10.03	13.03	9.90	8.71
Greece	7.63	10.38	11.72	14.97	9.54	12.53	11.66	11.65	14.83	12.63	8.51
Germany	16.49	14.16	12.66	11.94	12.14	10.02	12.96	13.12	12.12	12.94	7.78
Slovenia	16.17	14.99	13.91	14.08	15.67	11.94	12.81	8.72	9.89	14.67	7.53
Poland	17.47	12.66	15.22	14.95	17.45	12.76	11.26	13.54	13.25	16.02	6.92
Canada	13.88	17.32	16.57	15.13	15.78	18.54	15.07	12.70	10.21	10.79	6.85
Estonia	0.00	0.00	0.00	66.67	11.59	11.55	16.52	19.46	16.77	13.69	6.40
Czech Rep-	18.37	18.55	15.27	15.74	18.58	15.82	13.56	11.65	16.58	13.42	6.35
U.S.	17.20	17.12	17.35	19.67	18.59	15.65	15.85	17.48	16.40	14.87	5.88
China	0.00	0.00	0.00	0.00	88.39	23.55	19.22	16.96	16.15	18.40	5.47
Slovak	22.22	21.35	18.86	26.32	21.28	14.74	13.76	13.31	14.66	18.70	5.40
India	0.00	0.00	86.01	21.88	17.42	19.03	19.28	16.04	17.04	15.54	4.71
Lithuania	0.00	73.10	28.03	25.23	22.09	19.51	28.19	16.57	17.83	19.29	4.00
Latvia	83.16	25.08	23.49	24.14	18.36	24.65	20.17	24.23	15.45	18.85	3.60

AP = Average Persistency.

Source: our computations on IMS Health, Copyright 2005.

Table V.6   Product turnover as a share of existing products, top 100 ATC4 classes, 1995-2004

	1995	1996	1997	1998	1999	2000	2001	2002	2003	2004	Avg.
					Product entry rate (%)						
U.S.	12.15	16.64	18.81	15.30	15.45	9.05	14.13	n.a.	11.00	12.29	*13.87*
Japan	8.46	n.a.	8.69	n.a.	8.11	9.63	8.60	9.46	n.a.	7.87	*8.69*
EU-15	9.12	9.53	9.15	11.78	11.07	10.62	9.41	9.98	10.28	10.71	*10.17*
EU-25	9.30	9.54	9.33	11.91	11.11	10.67	9.46	10.00	10.31	10.65	*10.23*
					Product exit rate (%)						
U.S.	13.39	7.51	7.44	6.25	8.38	13.43	6.87	7.61	6.09	6.37	*8.33*
Japan	5.49	4.88	6.52	5.66	7.09	7.45	5.38	7.06	5.41	4.24	*5.92*
EU-15	n.a.	4.92	4.51	4.29	4.60	4.03	3.87	4.04	4.66	5.39	*4.48*
EU-25	n.a.	4.92	4.57	4.38	4.64	4.15	4.11	4.17	4.68	n.a.	*4.45*
					Product turnover (%)						
U.S.	25.54	24.14	26.25	21.55	23.84	22.47	21.00	n.a.	17.10	18.66	*22.28*
Japan	13.94	n.a.	15.21	n.a.	15.20	17.08	13.98	16.52	n.a.	12.11	*14.86*
EU-15	n.a.	14.44	13.66	16.07	15.67	14.65	13.28	14.02	14.94	16.10	*14.76*
EU-25	n.a.	14.46	13.91	16.29	15.76	14.82	13.57	14.17	15.00	n.a.	*14.75*
					Product net entry (%)						
U.S.	-1.24	9.13	11.37	9.05	7.07	-4.38	7.26	n.a.	4.91	5.92	*5.45*
Japan	2.97	n.a.	2.17	n.a.	1.02	2.18	3.22	2.40	n.a.	3.63	*2.51*
EU-15	n.a.	4.61	4.64	7.49	6.47	6.59	5.54	5.94	5.62	5.32	*5.80*
EU-25	n.a.	4.62	4.76	7.53	6.47	6.52	5.35	5.83	5.63	n.a.	*5.84*

n.a. correspond to computed entry and exit rates outside the range of average turnover +/- two times the standard deviation.

Source: our computations on IMS Health, Copyright 2005.

the penetration, in terms of quantities, on the market by generic producers is larger in the U.S. market (33.67 percent of the market in 2004) as compared to the European markets (volume share in EU-15 is 16.34 percent in 2004) and to Japan (see Table V.8). Among the European markets, only the Netherlands and UK show a level of generic penetration that resembles that of the U.S., respectively 39.99 percent and 31.01 percent in terms of volume (see Table A.V.1).

Generic products are sold at lower prices relative to the branded products that are available on the market. Table V.9 reports price

Table V.7   Market share of local non-multinational companies (non-MNCs)

Country	MS %	Country	MS %	Country	MS %	Country	MS %
Sweden	0.3	Finland	1.2	EU-25	3.7	Greece	9.8
Ireland	0.6	Austria	1.6	EU-15	3.7	Portugal	11.1
Belgium	0.9	Netherlands	2.6	Germany	4.3	Japan	17.1
UK	1.0	France	3.1	Spain	5.0	India	43.7
Denmark	1.1	U.S.	3.5	Italy	6.5	China	69.5

Source: our computations on IMS Health, Copyright 2005.

ratios for all pharmaceutical products, distinguishing brand-names and unbranded generics.[4] Prices have been converted in purchasing power parity (PPP) U.S. dollars. The average prices of branded drugs in the U.S. are almost double the corresponding prices in EU countries. EU average price for branded drugs is 50.7 percent of the U.S. level. However, generic drug prices in the EU-15 countries are 110.4 percent their U.S. counterparts.

After having adjusted prices for PPP, average prices of branded products in the EU-15 are 45.01 percent of the U.S. prices, whereas generic prices in EU-15 are 91.44 percent the U.S. price. More than half of the molecules included in the sample are priced higher in the U.S. than in any country of the EU-15.

Price differences between the U.S. and EU-15 are entirely explained by differences in prices of branded drugs. In fact, prices of generic drugs in the U.S. are substantially aligned with prices in EU-15. In a few countries, such as Germany, generic prices are higher than in the U.S.[5]

Table V.10 takes a different perspective and compares the price at launch of products introduced between 1994 and 2004, with the average prices of existing products in each country within the same ATC4 class. Price at entry of branded drugs is 43.4 percent higher in the U.S. than the prevailing average price in the market. The corresponding price gap in the EU-15 is 28.2 percent, and in Japan just 3.9 percent

---

[4] The data only allow us to distinguish branded products (both originator or licensee products and branded generics) from unbranded products, referred to in the table as "generics".

[5] However, in Germany generics are mostly "branded generics" rather than pure generics. These are included among the "branded" products.

Table V.8   Generic penetration in main regional markets, 1994-2004

Country	Sales (%)			Quantity (SU %)		
	1994	1999	2004	1994	1999	2004
U.S.	7.10	5.26	6.35	21.41	27.94	33.67
EU-15	3.41	4.25	8.69	7.61	9.89	16.34
EU-25	3.54	4.37	8.45	8.73	10.77	16.01
Japan	3.69	2.52	1.89	3.07	2.49	2.55

Source: our computations on IMS Health, Copyright 2005.

(see Table V.10). U.S. generic products, by contrast, enter at prices at 60.3 percent of the average prices in the market.

These price differentials between the U.S. and Europe reflect radical differences in the extent of market regulation.[6] Prices of branded drugs in countries with free or semi-regulated prices—such as the U.S. and, to a lesser extent, UK and Germany—are higher than in countries where more direct forms of price regulation are in place, such as Italy and France. At the same time, the relatively unregulated markets tend to experience fierce price competition after patent expiry, since higher prices of branded drugs represent a strong incentive for generic entry and price competition *à la Bertrand* (Pammolli *et al*, 2002; Magazzini *et al.* 2004).

Price convergence is taking place in Europe, as a combined effect of regulation at the level of single member states, parallel trade, and external reference pricing.

In order to shed light into this issue we compared prices in each EU-25 country considered in the analysis with the prices in EU-15 countries where molecules are available. The median of the price ratios for each country considered is reported in Figure V.4. The Figure shows that EU prices are converging toward a common mean. Convergence was more rapid in the second half of the 1990s as a result of the process of EU monetary convergence.

Germany is characterized by higher prices than the EU-15 countries, with a median price gap in 2004 equal to 20 percent. Although

---

[6] For an in-depth analysis of institutional aspects of national pharmaceutical markets, see OECD (2001).

Table V.9   Average molecule prices per Standard Unit, 2004
(U.S. = 100)

Country	Exchange rate			Parity Purchase Power[1]		
	All products	Generics	Branded	All products	Generics	Branded
Austria	60.17	149.81	44.64	54.61	136.57	40.64
Belgium	58.01	150.74	43.43	51.15	133.20	38.37
Canada	67.00	117.44	56.32	71.48	125.12	60.26
China	16.97	14.59	20.46	79.26	68.12	95.54
Czech Rep.	37.16	69.16	28.33	65.02	120.90	49.39
Denmark	61.93	105.16	48.14	45.28	77.32	35.22
Estonia	44.79	101.00	34.45	84.67	191.11	65.23
Finland	56.60	152.08	44.97	46.49	125.13	37.26
France	53.25	125.48	40.39	46.05	108.11	34.98
Germany	75.83	139.42	58.61	67.05	122.96	51.56
Greece	44.06	69.67	34.29	48.61	76.78	37.50
Hungary	39.64	97.85	27.61	61.46	154.23	42.85
India	14.56	13.37	10.34	22.77	20.86	15.90
Ireland	57.76	108.30	44.94	48.65	91.11	37.51
Italy	55.68	127.30	40.47	54.34	123.93	39.20
Japan	65.31	96.00	44.62	52.67	77.95	35.91
Latvia	41.29	86.22	31.66	90.56	189.33	69.40
Lithuania	40.22	62.94	32.19	80.10	125.78	64.14
Luxembourg	61.19	175.11	44.73	59.27	170.96	43.41
Netherlands	59.53	112.30	48.96	48.49	90.98	40.15
Poland	35.86	35.59	30.53	68.02	68.42	58.27
Portugal	53.20	152.55	38.82	60.44	174.08	43.95
Slovak Rep.	36.61	56.69	27.63	70.24	109.52	53.60
Slovenia	64.24	188.65	45.46	84.40	250.83	60.24
Spain	43.94	91.65	33.12	43.60	90.92	33.00
Sweden	64.46	109.97	50.21	49.34	84.89	38.76
UK	60.55	115.25	48.31	48.73	93.74	39.17
EU-15	62.85	110.37	50.70	55.75	91.44	45.01
EU-25	60.65	102.24	48.01	58.11	91.34	46.68

Source: our computations on IMS Health, Copyright 2005. Parity Purchase Power from IMF.

Table V.10 The ratio between drug price at launch and the mean price of branded drugs in the market, 1994-2004[1]

	Branded	Generics		Branded	Generics
Austria	1.220	0.836	Japan	1.039	0.820
Belgium	1.181	0.659	Portugal	1.162	0.777
Finland	1.253	0.855	Spain	1.550	0.703
France	1.339	0.769	Sweden	1.437	0.793
Germany	1.061	0.735	UK	1.410	0.873
Italy	1.248	0.827	U.S.	1.434	0.603
			EU15[1]	1.282	0.776

(1) Weighted average over all ATC4 classes for available countries.

Source: our computations on IMS Health, Copyright 2005.

rapidly converging to the mean, Denmark also has prices that are on average higher than EU-15 prices. In the case of the Netherlands, the price gap was significantly reduced over the period 1994-1997.

Not surprisingly, given the characteristics of its external reference pricing system, within the European Union, Greece is characterized by the lowest prices among the EU-15 countries. Also in Spain prices are on average lower than the EU-15, as an effect of tight control on pharmaceutical product pricing.

The bulk of other EU countries have prices which, on average, are aligned with the EU-15 average. Rapid convergence also characterizes the new EU member states, which almost filled the price gap over the last decade.

Table V.11 confirms the main evidence in Figure V.4 by reporting some descriptive statistics of the coefficient of variation of the price ratios.[7] On average the coefficient of variation is decreasing over time for the European countries, pointing to a reduced variation of price ratio within each country, i.e. convergence of prices across countries.

Next, Figure V.5 summarizes some key indicators for branded and generic products' life-cycle during the 20 years after a product's

---

[7] The coefficient of variation is computed by taking, within each country the ratio of the standard deviation and the average value of the price ratios that lie within the range defined by the 5th and the 95th percentile of the distribution.

Figure V.4   Pharmaceutical price convergence in EU25, 1994-2004*

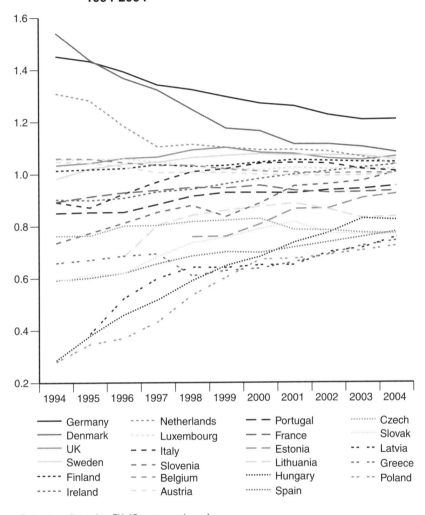

—— Germany	----- Netherlands	— — Portugal	········· Czech
—— Denmark	----- Luxembourg	— — France	········· Slovak
——— UK	- - - Italy	——— Estonia	-- -- Latvia
—— Sweden	- - - Slovenia	········ Lithuania	-- -- Greece
----- Finland	- - - Belgium	········ Hungary	-- -- Poland
----- Ireland	— — Austria	········ Spain	

*Country median price. EU-15 average price = 1.

Source: our computations on IMS Health, Copyright 2005.

launch in the U.S., Japan and main EU markets.[8] Except for the UK showing a flatter distribution of branded drug sales, the peak year of sales for branded drugs is found within five years from product's launch followed by a steep and prolonged decline. For generic products the profile is similar, although the sales distribution appears flat-

Table V.11   Descriptive statistics of the countries' coefficient of variation of price ratios, 1994-2004

	1994	1995	1996	1997	1998	1999	2000	2001	2002	2003	2004	CAGR
Min	.608	.605	.590	.567	.540	.514	.510	.522	.526	.520	.514	-1.67%
25th percentile	.656	.652	.644	.619	.606	.591	.581	.572	.558	.555	.549	-1.76%
Mean	.740	.731	.714	.690	.667	.641	.628	.619	.604	.599	.595	-2.15%
Median	.719	.716	.702	.706	.666	.643	.618	.602	.591	.585	.571	-2.27%
75th percentile	.805	.785	.785	.739	.720	.694	.678	.661	.629	.620	.619	-2.59%
Max	.905	.907	.850	.845	.799	.735	.730	.751	.737	.735	.745	-1.93%

Source: our computations on IMS Health, Copyright 2005

ter in Europe. This is straightforward since branded products face tougher competition especially after their patent expires,[9] while generics compete on the markets since their launch, therefore making the profile of their sales more evenly distributed. In the U.S., generic products also have a short life, with the majority of sales squeezed in the first years after launch.

Overall, faster diffusion of both branded and generic products characterizes the U.S., as compared to the European countries. Also price dynamics are markedly different when comparing European countries with the U.S. and Japan.

The time evolution of prices for branded drugs displays a substantial stability in the majority of EU countries compared to a marked increase in the U.S. (see the graph at the bottom left in Figure V.5). Prices of branded products in the U.S. constantly grow over time, being 30 percent higher with respect to launch after twenty years. On the contrary, branded prices in Germany, UK, and France are remarkably stable over time. Among the European countries, Italy is an exception, where branded prices start to increase few years after launch and are about 20 percent higher after 20 years. Japan is characterized by a different dynamic, where branded prices decrease over time and equal to 70 percent of launch price after 20 years.

In the U.S. prices of generic products fall sharply soon after launch (see the graph at the bottom right in Figure V.5). High competition on

---

[8] Years elapsed from launch are reported on the x-axis, whereas the y-axis report value, volume and price variations over the life cycle of pharmaceutical products.

[9] They face competition also by other molecules entering the same ATC4 class.

the off-patent segment of the market characterizes the U.S., where generic drug prices fall sharply soon after launch and volume and sales values are rapidly eroded.

The European scenario is quite mixed. On the one side, generic drug prices in Germany remain substantially stable over time. In France, prices remain stable in the first 8 years after launch. Then, prices fall towards a new stable path about 10 percent lower than the price at launch. In Italy, generic prices decrease soon after launch and then stabilize around 85 percent of price at launch.

Japanese prices of generic products continuously decrease over time, being 60 percent lower than the price at launch after 20 years.

Differences in price dynamics over the product life cycle unveil some key properties of market settings. In the unregulated U.S. market, innovative drugs can command large increases in prices during their lifetime. After patent expiry, they find it more profitable to charge high prices on a shrinking market share ("brand loyalty") rather than entering in price competition with generic manufacturers. On the other hand, generic drugs cannot count on innovativeness and/or brand loyal customers to promote their sales and therefore they engage in a fierce price competition *à la Bertrand*.

Conversely, in the EU, price regulation compresses margins on patented drugs, and their price differential with generic drugs is much lower than in the U.S. As a result, there is less segmentation between branded drugs and generic drugs, making the former important competitors for the latter.

This analysis of product life cycles confirms that the U.S. market is the most competitive, leading to faster renewal of products than in other markets. The unregulated price structure seems to play an important role in this process, by giving the appropriate incentives for the introduction of innovative drugs and the subsequent price competition between generic products that quickly displaces existing market shares.

Differences in price regulation across countries also explain why we observe a delay in the launch of new molecules in the EU with respect to the U.S. (see Figure V.5). In general, pharmaceutical companies tend to accelerate product launches in those markets where new products can be sold at a better price, in order to obtain the highest return to R&D expenditures and other fixed costs. (see Figure V.6).

Figure V.5   Product life cycles of branded (left) and generic (right) drugs:
a) distribution of sales in quantity (lifetime total = 1);
b) distribution of sales in value (lifetime total = 1);
c) price dynamics (launch date price = 1)

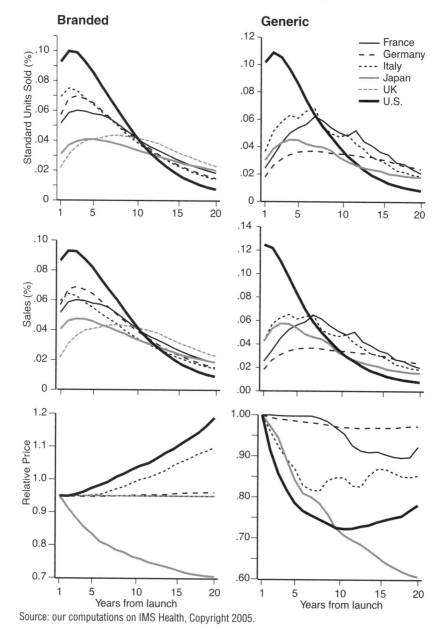

Source: our computations on IMS Health, Copyright 2005.

With the exception of the Netherlands, where the median launch is concomitant with the launch in the U.S., the European countries experience a time lag in the launch of new molecules. In the case of EU-15,[10] the median launch is delayed by eight months, while the delay increases to 17 months if we look at the EU-25. Overall, the delay is larger when comparing the launch in the U.S. with the launch in New Member States. Launch in Japan is further delayed with respect to Europe, having a median delay with respect to the U.S. of more than two years.

Differences in launch times between European countries and the U.S. and between countries within European are consistent with the price differentials discussed above and the results reported in the empirical literature, where the more strongly regulated countries were found to experience longer delay in new drug access (Danzon et al, 2003; Lanjouw, 2005; Kyle, 2006).

The entry lag in European markets of new molecules with respect to the U.S. is also influenced by the issue of parallel trading from European countries with lower prices (Italy, France) to those with higher prices (UK, Germany) and towards the U.S. (see also Chapter III).[11]

Another prominent aspect of competition in the pharmaceutical industry is the pricing strategy of drugs at launch. This issue has raised public concerns especially in face of the relentless rise of health care costs in industrialized economies.

Apart from the comparison between U.S. and EU, Table V.10 shows a common characteristic across countries, that is that new branded drugs tend to display higher prices than those already available on the market.

On average, what we observe is that new branded drugs quote a price at entry which is higher than those set for products already available in the market. As a result, after entry the average price of drugs increases. However, according to economic theory we would expect

---

[10] When considering the European aggregate, the comparison is made between the median launch across the European countries and the launch in the U.S.

[11] Innovative producers can choose not to introduce their products in countries with low market prices, in order to avoid that exports from these countries could erode their margins worldwide. The effect of parallel trading between EU countries is stronger since it is legally allowed within EU, while parallel trade toward the U.S. is illegal and therefore its effect is weaker.

Figure V.6   Introduction lag (in months) from launch on the U.S. market*

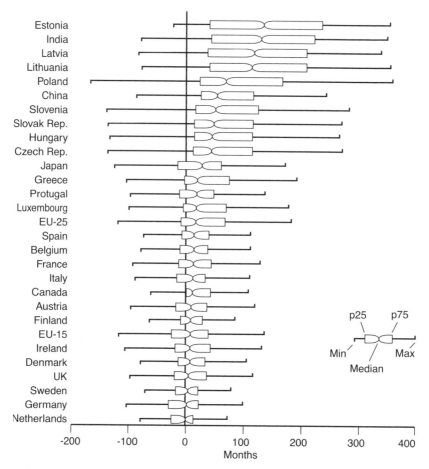

*All molecules commercialized both in the U.S. and selected countries since 1975. Outliers have been omitted. Positive values = months of delay from the U.S. launch. Negative values = months in advance as compared to the U.S. launch.

Source: our computations on IMS Health, Copyright 2005.

that entry leads to more competition and hence lower prices. How can be explained this puzzling evidence?

An important general discussion of new product pricing is due to Dean (1969), who considers two different strategies for new products, i.e. *skimming pricing* and *penetration pricing*. The former consists in setting an initial high price and then lowering it over time, while the latter lies in launching a new product at a low price and then raising it. According to Dean, skimming strategy is used for new products that offer significant advantages over existing one, while penetration pricing is more often employed for products representing only marginal improvements over their established competitors. Similar arguments are used by Reekie (1978) in his analysis of pricing of new pharmaceuticals, examining the initial prices of NME launched into the U.S. market between 1958 and 1975. He argues that, as a rule, new drugs representing important therapeutic advances are priced significantly above their existing substitutes, while imitators are priced much lower. Hence, Reekie concludes that new patented drugs have not limited price competition and in addition, he observes that over time drugs with higher prices tend to be subject of price reduction, while the opposite is true for new drugs with lower introductory prices. Like Reekie, Weston (1979, 1982) finds that higher launch prices can be often considered as premium prices for the quality upgrading embodied by new drugs with respect to the existing ones.

On the demand side another important aspect arises, that is the buyers' perception of a new product. Shapiro (1983) analyzes the optimal pricing strategy of firms taking into account the effect of imperfect buyer information on product characteristics for the so called "experienced goods", i.e. those whose characteristics can be ascertained after consumption. Setting up a monopoly model, Shapiro considers two cases. If consumers initially overestimate product quality, then the optimal pricing strategy for a firm is to "milk a reputation" through a high launch price followed by a declining path over time. On the contrary, if consumers underestimate products' characteristics the firm optimally decides to set a low price but intends to increase.

In the case of pharmaceutical industry, Lu *et al.* (1998) argue that competition often occurs among differentiated products with differing levels of buyer acceptance. Even under the assumption of horizontal differentiation, i.e. new drugs do not provide a significantly better quality than existing ones, the entrants' ability to attract buyers depends on how close their products are in terms of attributes to the existing ones. If they are neither identical nor too dissimilar, the best response of the incumbent product to entry could be to increase its price. In fact, the entry of new drugs with different characteristics from those already available on the market increases the consumer benefits due to enhanced matching between buyers' needs and product characteristics.

However, in the context of pharmaceuticals new drugs tend to attract more demand when their characteristics are preferred by a large number of consumers, which in general require that they provide substantial therapeutic benefits as compared to the existing products. Alternatively, if these products do not offer therapeutic improvement, consumers demand lower prices. This consideration suggests that more improved products will have higher introductory prices than their established competitors, while "me-too" or imitative products will not. In addition, in these cases higher launch prices tend to lower over time as the initial price premium will attract new potential rivals, so the originating firms will face increased competition in the future years. This argument also explains why a high market concentration, like the U.S. one, ultimately leads to a high turnover in sales.

Hence, high prices of new pharmaceuticals do not produce inflation dynamics if new branded products bring novel therapeutic benefits. In this case, reducing the premium price, through therapeutic reference pricing for patented products, lessen returns from innovation and hence incentives to invest in R&D.

In the near future this problem will be exacerbated by the arrival of new biopharmaceutical products on the market. Biopharmaceuticals are a class of therapeutic products produced by modern biotechnological techniques (recombinant DNA and hybridoma technology) that is to say therapeutic proteins synthesized in engineered biological systems. Second generation engineered biopharmaceuticals, especially humanized (since 1997) and human (since 2002) monoclonal antibodies, have provide new and effective therapies for cancer, cardiovascular disease, inflammatory diseases, macular degeneration, transplant rejection, and viral infection. In the case of biopharmaceuticals the definition of 'product' is inseparable from its production 'process' and manufacturing operation. This close linkage between 'product' and 'process' means there will not be a quick advent of low-cost alternatives or biogenerics and implies capacity-constraints. The increasing number of new biologicals, price and sales trends in a regime of production and regulatory constraints, raise serious concerns as far as future access, diffusion and sustainability of (bio)pharmaceutical innovation is concerned. First of all, a common definition of biopharmaceutical is strongly needed. Second, to ensure dynamic competition, it is important to favor off-patent competition (biogenerics, or biological follow-ons), within the jurisdiction of the FDA, EMEA and other national authorities, by establishing standards for approving biogenerics.[12]

In conclusion, the U.S. market for pharmaceuticals is both more concentrated and more dynamic than markets in Europe. Nonetheless, the higher concentration of the U.S. market does not mean that it is less competitive. On the contrary, the U.S. market is highly contestable; product turnover is much higher than in the EU and Japan; and competition from generic producers is substantial. The U.S. market regime is characterized by Schumpeterian competition, where innovators can gain temporary quasi-monopoly profits, which in turn spur innovation efforts by competitors. That quickly leads to more innovative products and a high turnover of market shares. The country with the least onerous market regulation shows also the highest renewal rate of products, thereby contributing to reduce the rents accruing to older products. Indeed, the U.S. market is characterized by the fastest market share erosion and price dynamics, corresponding to higher market mobility in price, quantities, and therefore total sales and market shares. Instead, dynamic competition is less evident in the EU as a whole, and especially in some continental and Mediterranean European countries.

---

[12] Biogenerics have already appeared in India, China, Latin America, and the Middle East.

Figure V.7   Biopharmaceutical products are gaining momentum: U.S. market share, relative price, number of products on the market and number of standard units sold.

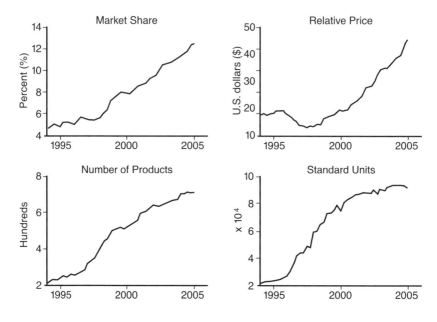

Appendix V

Appendix V.1

Table A.V.1   Generic penetration, 1994-2004

Country	Sales (%)			Quantities (Standard Units %)		
	1994	1999	2004	1994	1999	2004
U.S.	7.10	5.26	6.35	21.41	27.94	33.67
EU-15	3.41	4.25	8.69	7.61	9.89	16.34
EU-25	3.54	4.37	8.45	8.73	10.77	16.01
Japan	3.69	2.52	1.89	3.07	2.49	2.55
India	–	1.86	0.58	–	1.68	0.54
China	–	33.56	23.76	–	41.46	33.97
Canada	10.29	13.01	14.64	16.55	22.08	29.28
Czech Rep.	9.06	6.58	4.91	15.88	13.79	11.32
Estonia	–	12.52	6.35	–	27.79	19.95
Hungary	4.67	3.97	3.23	7.78	8.31	6.35
Latvia	–	16.27	8.17	–	24.40	22.27
Lithuania	–	13.36	7.14	–	27.43	23.56
Poland	13.59	7.59	5.28	28.58	22.43	16.24
Slovak Rep.	10.57	5.46	3.99	18.42	13.47	10.50
Slovenia	4.01	3.34	1.89	5.40	3.51	2.09
Austria	1.46	1.71	3.59	1.36	1.97	4.89
Belgium	0.90	1.13	5.29	1.32	2.55	9.65
Denmark	5.68	4.79	7.41	12.79	11.32	11.80
Finland	1.33	1.17	3.18	4.46	3.76	6.34
France	1.23	1.51	6.58	2.25	3.00	11.26
Germany	5.15	6.17	11.08	7.84	11.84	21.56
Greece	0.61	0.66	0.40	1.36	1.78	1.32
Ireland	1.83	1.40	0.50	5.74	5.23	2.56
Italy	0.95	0.69	2.55	1.09	1.06	5.07
Luxembourg	1.16	0.83	1.07	1.31	1.62	3.05
Netherlands	8.27	11.04	15.84	19.39	30.57	39.99
Portugal	1.01	1.83	8.47	0.44	0.80	7.18
Spain	1.80	2.28	5.25	3.15	3.65	9.08
Sweden	4.50	3.16	5.57	6.74	7.66	15.13
UK	8.02	10.81	18.66	24.40	26.77	31.01

Source: our computations on IMS Health, Copyright 2005.

Appendix V.2

Market Regulation, Innovation and Competition

To bring new compounds from the bench to the market firms must engage in expensive and risky R&D activities. As a consequence, the profit of pharmaceutical companies and improvements in social welfare depends, to a large extent, on the success of risky R&D efforts. The decision to sustain large sunk R&D costs critically depends upon the attrition rates of R&D projects and the expected market return from investment. In Chapter IV we have shown that attrition rates are increasing. Moreover, despite the fact that there are theoretical arguments and empirical evidence that a negative relationship exists between price regulation, dynamic competition and innovative efforts, most health care payers in both industrialized and less developed countries are understandably concerned about monopoly power and high prices of pharmaceuticals and, in most cases, have implemented explicit price controls and limits on the extent of patent rights. Taken together, the two effects raise serious concerns about growth and sustainability of innovation in the pharmaceutical industry.

While the cost of R&D is to a certain extent known, certain and rising, the probability of success and the market benefit π associated to R&D projects are to a large extent uncertain. For the sake of simplicity, we can assume that each firm knows the stochastic properties of market returns and aim at maximizing the expected present value of net benefits, with a discount rate that is hold constant. In other words, a successful project has an expected discounted payoff of π. If drug development is discontinued for some reason the expected payoff is L, the liquidation value of the compound if it does not hit the market. Let α be the probability of success and C the sunk cost of R&D. The first-best decision rule is to invest in the project provided that:

$$\alpha\pi - C \geq L$$

which is equivalent to $\pi \geq R/\alpha$, where $R = C + L$ is the total cost of R&D. The higher are total R&D expenditures and the probability of failure, the higher has to be the expected market returns in order to decide to undertake a given R&D project. Based on this simple relationship it is straightforward to notice that the market value has to be particularly high in the case of complex diseases and radically new therapeutic approaches. Moreover, as we have shown in Chapter IV, if α is decreasing and R is increasing, π has to increase in order to keep the same level of investment in R&D. Finally, it is evident that in most cases private incentives may not be sufficient to tackle orphan diseases.

At any given moment, a firm must decide whether to invest in R&D or to wait. If the current value of the project is above the critical threshold $\pi^* = R/\alpha$, the firm decides to invest. As a consequence, the "markup" $\pi^* - C$ reflects the value of waiting for more information. Due to the trade-off between larger versus later benefits, the optimal choice of π^* is that for which the additional net benefit from making π^* larger just balances the additional cost of discounting. Hence, some firms will undertake the most profitable R&D projects first and continue to undertake additional investment projects so long as the expected rate of return from the next project exceeds the firm's marginal cost of capital. Again, this is in line with the "fishing out" argument we raised in Chapter IV and the increasing complexity of pharmaceutical R&D. On the contrary, some firms will prefer to wait to license in compounds in a later stage of development and/or to engage in some form of "me-too" competition.

During the regime of patent protection, firms that successfully launched an innovative product benefit from an exclusive market position to charge higher prices ($\bar{p}$). Typically, drug patents provide strong protection against competition because analogous compounds must undergo all clinical trials request by the competent national authorities from the very beginning. In all industrialized countries with the important exception of the U.S., after patent expiry the price of drugs drastically drop to $\underline{p}$ due to the entry of generic drugs and *Bertrand* competition (Pammolli *et al.* 2002, Magazzini *et al.* 2004). However, it is generally true that patented drugs are able to rapidly capture the lion share of their therapeutic markets and outperform unpatented drugs in terms of sales in the first eight years after launch.

The actual extension of the regime of higher prices is unknown ex-ante and depends on regulatory interventions in single national markets (patent-term extension or reduction), international free-ridership, parallel trade and potential competitors, each of which is trying to develop its own patent. The success of a competitor might cause π to fall by some random amount. Over time, additional competitors may succeed in entering the market and governmental agencies should restrict the extent of patent rights, so that π continues to fall.[13] As a result, the expected value of a "sunk" cost investment can be obtained by summing up expected product revenues in the exclusive and competitive regimes.

Moreover, governmental agencies can implement explicit price control. These can take several forms, including capping the prices of new drugs at the level of prior substitute therapies and sometimes at the level of the lowest price substitute, allowing prices that are no higher than those levied for the same product in other "reference" nations and imposing on individual physicians annual budgets for drug expenditures, which if exceeded lead to fee reductions. All these regulatory interventions are aimed at reducing drug prices and price differentials $(\bar{p}-\underline{p})$. Arguably, production and marketing costs (A) as well as the elasticity of the demand (ε) are not directly affected by regulation.[14] Hence, the expected market returns π can be decomposed into two components corresponding to different market regimes:

$$\pi = \lambda(1-\delta)\overline{M} + (1-\lambda)(1-\delta)\underline{M} + \delta M^{R} - A$$

where λ is the proportion of the final market in which firms are granted market power (for a given period) by patent protection, δ is the proportion of the final market subject to price regulation, $\overline{M} > M^{R} > \underline{M}$ are the share of market payoffs under different regimes, and A is the total marketing and production cost. In the U.S. case δ is almost zero so market competition regimes are split in two: quasi-monopolistic pricing/high profits pre-patent expiry and *Bertrand* competition/low profits after patent expiry. On the contrary in Europe δ is almost one. Stronger patent protection regime and looser price regulation in absence of parallel trade and spillovers among markets regimes shall lead to higher expected market returns as the company can sustain higher prices in a larger share of the final market and for a longer time period.

---

[13] The calculation of the investment in this case turns out to be extremely difficult. In the next session we apply a numerical solution method to take into account the effect of competition on investment decisions.

[14] The pharmaceutical market is characterized by a price-inelastic demand mainly due to extensive medical insurance. Since individuals, once they are ill, only pay a small fraction of their medical costs, prices are likely to have a limited effect. This does not only affect the choice of whether or not to consume a drug, but also the choice between alternative drug treatments.

As a consequence, both price and patent regulation contributes to lower incentives to sustain sunk cost investments in R&D which could speed up the passage to the threshold (π^*). Companies are likely to take into account the effect of regulation in their future investment decisions. As a result, pharmaceutical firms would either reduce or postpone "sunk" R&D investments. Moreover, in the presence of an international reference price scheme (such as the European mean price) it can be easily demonstrated that it is rational to delay product launches in countries with a regulated market regime M^R characterized by lower prices and/or weaker patent protection after having introduced a new compound in countries that ensure an higher price ($\overline{M}$).

Based on the market settings described so far, we have tested the impact of price and patent regulation on the pharmaceutical entry, competition and firm turnover by means of a simulative exercise. Namely, we evaluate the effects of a generalized five percent price cut and a 15 percent patent term reduction.[15] Let $S_i(t)$ be total sales of firm i at time t. Total sales at the firm level are obtained by summing up product sales figures:

$$S_i(t) = \sum_j s_{i,j}(t)$$

where $s_{i,j}(t)$ correspond to the sales of product j of firm i at time t.

The product and firm's growth on yearly basis are computed as follows:

Product sales growth: $G_i(t) = S_i(t)/S_i(t-1)$

Firm sales growth: $g_{i,j}(t) = s_{i,j}(t)/s_{i,j}(t-1)$

Figure V.7 depicts the empirical probability distribution of product growth rates as obtained by computing the frequency of companies in fifty equally spaced groups of growth $G(t)$. Having fixed the empirical benchmark in terms of growth distributions, we are ready now to start our simulative exercise. We simulate a model of firm growth based on the following assumptions: (1) product market performances evolve according to a stochastic process of proportionate growth; (2) the

---

[15] The original version of the model was applied to estimate the effect of the Italian Decree DL 15/04/2002, no. 63 on pharmaceutical expenditure containment (Pammolli *et al.*, 2002).

probability that the next market opportunity (a new product) is filled by any currently active firm is proportional to the number of products of that firm.

Innovative efforts are modeled at the product level as departures from a process of proportionate growth. After launch, performances of patented drugs exceed market performances of non-patented products. For a short period of time (2-3 years) they grow more than proportionally to their size. After this period of sustained growth they start to converge slowly to the mean rate of growth at the market level. For patented products we set more than proportional growth till patent expiry and a less than proportional growth afterward. The two parts of patented product lifecycle correspond to the regime of high prices ($\overline{M}$) and low prices ($\underline{M}$) respectively. Based on such assumptions, we simulate the market evolution of products. Successively, products are randomly assigned to companies according to a proportional allocation rule (Ijiri an Simon, 1977). At each time step, new products are drawn and assign to companies in proportion to the number of products they already have. We have demonstrated in a previous work that this process perfectly fit the actual distribution of the number of products by company, the as well as the growth and size distribution of products and companies (De Fabritiis *et al.*, 2003, Fu *et al.*, 2005, Buldyrev *et al.* 2007, Growiec *et al.* 2007).

In short, our simulation runs in two steps: first, product sales performances are generated according to a proportionate growth process, then products are randomly assign to companies in proportion to the number of products they have. The growth distributions generated by our simulation are also reported in Figure V.7. First we consider a basic setting of the simulation parameter that accurately fit the real distribution (dotted lines). Afterwards the two effects discussed above are introduced. Assuming an inelastic demand, the five percent price cut is simulated as a corresponding reduction of firm sales (light gray lines).[16] The patent term reduction is simulated by reducing the expiry time for patented products (dark gray lines). As a last simulation, we combined the two measures together (heavy black lines). Both the measures considered significantly reduce market turnover.

---

[16] The absence of co-payment mechanisms seems to support such an assumption of indifference of customers to price chances.

Figure A.V.1   Pharmaceutical firms' growth distribution (real data 1994-2004) and the effect of price and patent regulation (simulation results)

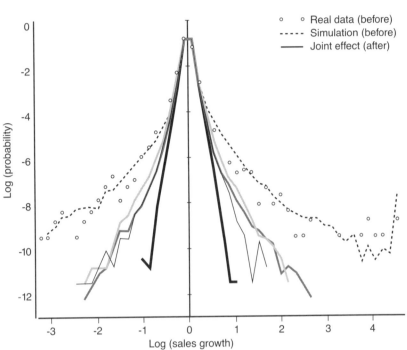

Source: our computations on IMS Health, Copyright 2005.

All in all, price regulation and patent term reduction reduce firm mobility, and episodes of highly positive (and negative) sales performances are deemed to become more and more unlikely. In synthesis, price and patent regulation is likely to reduce (or postpone) firm turnover, incentives to invest in R&D and to entry the market with vertically differentiated products. In a regulated market regime, it is likely to observe horizontal differentiation strategies to delay or avoid relevant investments in R&D (co-marketing licenses and imitative behavior), and collusive conducts, with negative effects on market competition and productivity.

In a nutshell, we have identified two effects of regulation on the degree of innovation and competitiveness of the pharmaceutical industry.

First, generalized price ceilings and cuts will probably reduce incentives to sustain sunk cost investments, inducing firms to postpone their decisions in order to collect more information and signals on the future regulatory agenda (i.e. through co-marketing licenses and imitative strategies). On the contrary, alternative measures such as an enforcement of market-like mechanisms after patent expiry though the introduction of generic products and/or a price cut of old drugs to favor the entry of new medicines (market regime $\underline{M}$) would not affect the "price-premium" for innovation and the incentive to sunk cost investments.

Second, patent term contraction and limitation to the extent of patent rights penalize innovative efforts and dynamic competition. Whereas frequently patented medicines are subject to both price caps and limitation to the extent of patent rights, unpatented drugs of the same generation are affected only by price containment. Moreover, it is useful to note that rational adaptive agents would take into consideration the risk of future regulatory intervention in their investment and drug launch decisions.

Chapter VI
Conclusions

Chapter VI

Conclusions

The European pharmaceutical industry was one of the great post-war success stories, with Europe outpacing the United States. The evidence presented in this volume has documented the relative decline of European countries and firms in the last 25 years, and reforms that are needed if Europe is to recover and to return to achieve higher rates of growth and higher productivity levels.

Research and Innovation

Despite a positive trade balance of the EU with respect to the U.S. in recent years, European countries lag behind the U.S. in research and development activities.

The disappointing performance of Europe as a location for R&D activities in pharmaceuticals mirrors what we observe of the leading forces spurring productivity growth.

In Europe total factor productivity growth has not been accompanied by capital accumulation. Since capital accumulation also captures physical investments in R&D, such a trend casts doubts on the sustainability of the EU growth model, especially if we consider that China and India are accumulating scientific and technological capabilities in the life sciences and in pharmaceuticals, moving to a more knowledge intensive development pattern.

This evolution, which is sustained also by the emergence of high skill "diaspora networks" centered in the U.S., poses a serious challenge to the European pharmaceutical industry, which might be displaced in the long run by economies with skilled human capital, lower labor costs, and greater potential in terms of both market size and scientific capabilities.

The internal structure of the U.S. national innovation system is a powerful source of competitive advantage and industrial leadership. In the U.S. the biotech sector play a vital role integrating explorations of new research opportunities with clinical and market development. On the contrary, Europe suffers a lack of dynamism of young technology-dedicated firms generating and developing R&D projects. In this context, too little attention has been devoted so far to the important role of institutional investors and capital markets in sustaining the development and growth of a European biotechnology industry.

Market Regulation Regimes

So far, efforts aimed at developing a Single Market for pharmaceuticals have failed. Regulation and the heterogeneity of pricing and reimbursement schemes, as well as cost containment policies in Europe had a negative effect on the upstream innovation phase of the drug industry as well as on the downstream stage relating to the launch of innovative drugs. To achieve better productivity performance, the level of competitive intensity must be increased in Europe, fully opening the European markets to global competition, achieving a higher level of integration in medical services, and reforming distribution channels to achieve higher levels of efficiency through market competition.

At present, marketing authorization is restricted by complex evaluations of new drugs applications that differ across European countries. Although there has been a gradual move towards harmonization of regulatory standards with the Mutual Recognition and the Centralized Procedures, pharmaceutical companies must still negotiate with individual countries over price whichever regulatory route is used. Cross country differences in price regulation delay the launch of innovative products, as they encourage arbitrage by wholesalers across different markets with a detrimental effect on incentives to innovation. This in turn affects the attractiveness of the EU for R&D investments, since an excessive pressure on R&D returns can contribute to high value added activities and R&D moving to other, more dynamic, markets. Hence, the administrative and regulatory integration of the European pharmaceutical market has to be considered a priority for the competitiveness of the European drug industry.

U.S. pharmaceutical prices have been more than double the EU-15 average in the past decade. Branded drugs account for this gap, while prices of generic drugs are in line with the EU-15 average. In Europe less regulated markets such as the United Kingdom and Germany display higher prices than countries like France and Italy, which rely upon price regulation systems. U.S. prices of generic drugs are substantially aligned with the EU-15 average, and in many cases they are well below European and Canadian prices for generics.

More extensive generic prescribing and use of relatively less expensive generics in the United States has fostered a competitive generics market there, and has helped to free up financial resources that are used in turn to fund greater consumption of innovative drugs by patients for whom those medicines constitute the most appropriate and beneficial treatment option. By artificially constraining prices of innovative medicines while failing to stimulate a robust and competitive market for generic medicines, European governments are missing the opportunity to create "headroom" for innovation.

Transatlantic Dialogue

The uneven geographical distribution of research activities in pharmaceuticals, together with the observed differences in price levels for innovative drugs and in reimbursement schemes between Europe and the U.S., as well as across European countries, call for a revival of transatlantic dialogue on the political economy of the pharmaceutical industry, with particular reference to trade policy and the protection of intellectual property rights.

Such a dialogue is particularly important, at a time in which policy makers are struggling to balance the goals of encouraging and rewarding innovation while keeping it affordable.

In the long run, for both Europe and the U.S., industrial productivity, as well as the role and direction of pharmaceutical innovation, will be affected by the interplay between technological advances and patterns of demand, especially in relation to the effective management of health and pharmaceutical expenditures to encourage innovation while preserving the fiscal sustainability of national health systems.

Data for most recent years show, for the first time, a slowdown in total factor productivity (TFP) growth for the U.S. Such a negative result comes from a combination of an upsurge of the level of investment, delay in the production of measurable output from past R&D, and decline in market growth rates for existing products. This result, if confirmed in the upcoming years, could be the first sign of an imbalance, and could not be sustained without further consolidation and/or lower R&D effort.

Health care financing

A significant fraction of EU health care is tax funded: healthy young workers pay for the care of sick, usually older and poorer citizens. In turn, young generations rely on future generations to pay for their care. But demographic changes—a falling birth rate and growing life expectancy—are likely to cause severe funding problems within the existing framework, which will worsen over the years.

According to the most recent European Commission (EPC) projections, spending on public health care and long-term care in the EU will grow by 2.2 percent of GDP by 2050, moving from 7.3 to 9.4 percent of GDP. This represents a 30 percent increase—and it may be a serious underestimate (De la Dehesa, 2006; Pammolli and Salerno, 2006).

The official projections assume a remarkably optimistic set of hypotheses about future economic and demographic developments. Unemployment rates in every country are assumed to fall beneath their recent historical average, which is unlikely without radical labor market reforms. Furthermore, the official projections assume that fertility rates will rise in most developed countries, with the highest percentage increases in those countries that currently have the lowest rates.

In many European countries, government programs to finance health and pharmaceuticals have displaced private efforts and private insurance programs, preventing the establishment of a price mechanism capable to account for physicians and consumer preferences, by which individuals can indicate their preferences and their willingness.

This status quo does not contribute to the efficiency of health care and pharmaceutical delivery and financing. On the contrary, the total level of health spending and its allocation among different services and products tend to perpetuate historic patterns of care and consumption, instead of responding to the preferences of European people.

The presence of multiple institutional investors and organizations that enter into contractual arrangements with health care providers and pharmaceutical companies would meet the diverse preferences of consumers, offering greater variety and more flexible health care plans. Multiple buyer systems have sometimes been criticized as a factor responsible for the increased price of health care in the U.S. However, in Europe, the introduction of multiple buyer systems as a complement to the current public programs might attenuate the perverse effects on health care expenditure caused by over-consumption of products and services under public insurance programs.

Against this background, a key point of reference for European governments should be the recognition of the uncertainty inherent in biomedical and pharmaceutical research, as well as the heterogeneity of individual attitudes and preferences.

We believe that both in Europe and in the U.S. the key challenge for governments is how to design pluralistic systems of health care delivery and financing, in which market forces can act to promote competition and so generate an environment favorable to investment and innovation, while public and private programs can combine to make patterns of care responsive to individual preferences without imposing excessive financial burdens on individuals or denying necessary care because of inability to pay (Feldstein, 1995).

Institutional reforms to sustain a competitive environment

The disappointing performance of the European pharmaceutical industry cannot be fully explained by sector-specific factors. It is also the consequence of Europe's relative lack of dynamism in introducing horizontal reforms aimed at improving the overall business environment as well as reforming its labor and capital markets, education systems, public spending, and regimes of market regulation (Alesina and Giavazzi, 2006).

It is only by combining sector-specific actions and broad market oriented reforms of economic institutions that Europe can generate a predictable and attractive business environment. Transforming the European institutional and business environment is a necessity if Europe aims at increasing productivity and promoting job creation in high value added, science based industries like pharmaceuticals.

References

Acemoglu D. and J. Linn (2004), "Market Size in Innovation: Theory and Evidence from the Pharmaceutical Industry," *The Quarterly Journal of Economics*, 119(3), 1049-1090.

Aghion P. and P. Howitt (1992), "A Model of Growth Through Creative Destruction," *Econometrica*, 60 (2) 323-351.

Aghion P. and P. Howitt (1998a), "Market structure and the growth process," *Review of Economic Dynamics*, 1, 276-305.

Aghion P. and P. Howitt (1998b), "On the Macroeconomic effects of Major Technological Change" in Helpman, E., Ed., *General Purpose Technologies and Economic Growth*, Cambridge, MA: MIT Press.

Aghion P. and R. Griffith (2005), *Competition and Growth*, Cambridge, MA: MIT Press.

Ahn S. (2002), "Competition, Innovation And Productivity Growth: A Review Of Theory And Evidence," Economics Department Working Papers No. 317.

Aitken B.J. and A.E. Harrison (1999), "Do Domestic Firms Benefit from Direct Foreign Investment? Evidence from Venezuela," *The American Economic Review*, 89(3), 605-618.

Alesina, A., S. Ardagna, G. Nicoletti and F. Schiantarelli (2005), "Regulation and Investment," *Journal of European Economic Association*, 3, 791-825.

Alesina A., E. Spolaore, and R. Wacziarg (2003), "Trade, Growth and the Size of Countries," Chap. 23, *Handbook of Economic Growth*, 1(2), 1499-1542.

Amercham Belgium (2002), "US Direct Investment in Belgium 2001/2002," The American Chamber of Commerce in Belgium, Brussels.

Anderson J.H. (1979), "A Theoretical Foundation for the Gravity Equation," *American Economic Review*, 69, 106-116.

Alesina A., and F. Giavazzi (2006), *The Future of Europe. Reform or Decline*, Cambridge MA: MIT Press.

Altshuler, R., H. Grubert and T. S. Newlon (1998), *Has U.S. investment abroad become more sensitive to tax rates?* Cambridge MA: NBER Working Paper 6383.

Ark B. van, R. Inklaar, and R. McGuckin (2002), "Changing Gear—Productivity, ICT and Services Industries: Europe and the United States," GGDC Research Memorandum GD-60.

Arora A. and A. Gambardella (1994a), "Explaining Technological Information and Utilizing it: Scientific Knowledge, Capacity, and External Linkages in Biotechnology," *Journal of Economic Behavior and Organization*, 24, 91-114.

Arora A. and A. Gambardella (1994b), "The Changing Technology of Technical Change: General and Abstract Knowledge and the Division of Innovative Labour," *Research Policy*, 23, 523-532.

Arora A. and A. Gambardella (2006), *From Underdogs to Tigers: The Rise and Growth of the Software Industry in Brazil, China, India, Ireland, and Israel*, Oxford University Press.

Arora A., A. Gambardella, F. Pammolli, and M. Riccaboni (2000), "The Nature and the Extent of the Market for Technology in Biopharmaceuticals," paper presented at the International Conference on Technology Policy and Innovation, Paris.

Arora, A., A. Fosfuri, and A. Gambardella (2001), *Markets for Technology*, Cambridge, MA: MIT Press.

Athreye S., and D. Kale (2006): "Experimentation With Strategy in the Indian Pharmaceutical Sector," Paper presented at the International Schumpeterian Society Conference, 2006.

Barba Navaretti G. and A.J. Venables (2004), *Multinational Firms in the World Economy*, Princeton University Press.

BEA (2006), *International Economic Accounts*, Bureau of Economic Analysis, Washington.

Begg D. (1998), "Pegging Out: Lessons from the Czech Exchange Rate Crisis," *Journal of Comparative Economics*, 26(4), 669-690.

Berndt E. R. (2001), "The U.S. Pharmaceutical Industry: Why Major Growth in Times of Cost Containment?" *Health Affairs*, 20(2), 100-114.

Berndt E. R. (2002), "Pharmaceuticals in the U.S. Healthcare: Determinants of Quantity and Price," *Journal of Economic Perspectives*, 14(4), 45-66.

Berndt E. R., Busch A.M., Frank R. G. (2007), "Medicare Part D, Prescription Drug Prices, and Treatment Quality," paper to be presented at the 2007 Annual Meetings of the American Economic Association, Chicago, Illinois.

Bergstrand, J.H. (1985), "The Generalized Gravity Equation, Monopolistic Competition, and the Factor-Proportions Theory in International Trade," *Review of Economics and Statistics*, 71, 143-153.

Bergstrand, J.H. (1989), "The Gravity Equation in International Trade: Some Microeconomic Foundations and Empirical Evidence," *Review of Economics and Statistics*, 67, 474-481.

Blanchard O. (1993), "Consumption and the Recession of 1990-1991," *American Economic Review*, 83(2), 270-74.

Blanchard O. (2002), "Comments on 'Catching up with the Leaders: The Irish Hare', by Patrick Honohan and Brendan Walsh," Brookings Papers of Economic Activity, 1, 58-66.

Blanchard O. (2004), "The Economic Future of Europe," *Journal of Economic Perspectives*, 18(4), 3-26.

Bresnahan, T. F., and M. Trajtenberg, (1996), "General Purpose Technologies: Engines of Growth?" *Journal of Econometrics*, Annals of Econometrics, 65, 83-108.

Buldyrev, S. V., J. Growiec, F. Pammolli, M. Riccaboni, H. E. Stanley (2007), "The Growth of Business Firms: Facts and Theory," *Journal of the European Economic Association*, 5 (2/3), forthcoming.

Chadha A. (2005), "TRIPS and Patenting Activity: Evidence from the Indian Pharmaceutical Industry," National University of Singapore, Department of Economics, Working Paper n.0512.

Chandler A.D. (2005), *The Remarkable Story of the Evolution of the Modern Chemical and Pharmaceutical Industries*, Cambridge, MA: Harvard University Press.

Chaudhuri S., Goldberg P.K., Gia P. (2006), "Estimating the Effects of Global Patent Protection in Pharmaceuticals: A Case Study of Quinolones in India," *American Economic Review*, 96(5).

Chen, D. (2000), "The Marginal Effective Tax Rate: The Only Tax Rate That Matters in Capital Allocation," C.D. Howe Institute Backgrounder. Toronto: C.D. Howe Institute

Cockburn I.M. (2004), "The Changing Structure of the Pharmaceutical Industry," *Health Affairs*, 23(1), 10-22.

Cockburn I. and J. Lanjouw (2001), "New pills for poor people? Empirical evidence after GATT," *World Development*, 29.

Cohen W., R. Nelson, and J. Walsh (2000), "Protecting Their Intellectual Assets: Appropriability Conditions and Why U.S. Manufacturing Firms Patent (or Not)," NBER Working Paper 7552.

Corsetti G., L. Dedola, and S. Leduc (2006), "Productivity, External Balance and Exchange Rates: Evidence on the Transmission Mechanism among G7 Countries," NBER Working Paper 12483.

CPB (2001), *Capital Income Taxation in Europe: Trends and Trade-offs*, The Hague, CPB.

Crepon B., Duguet E., Mairesse J. (1998), "Research, Innovation and Productivity: An Econometric Analysis at the Firm Level," NBER Working Paper 6696.

Criscuolo C. and R. Martin (2003), "Multinationals, and US productivity leadership: Evidence from Britain," London, UK: *CERIBA Discussion Paper*.

Danzon, P. (1998), "The Economics of Parallel Trade," *PharmacoEconomics*, 13(3), 293-304.

Danzon, P and L. Chao (2000), "Cross-national price differences for pharmaceuticals: how large, and why?" *Journal of Health Economics*, 19(2), 159-195.

Danzon P. and M.V. Pauly (2002), "Health Insurance and the Growth in Pharmaceutical Expenditures," *Journal of Law and Economics*, 45, 587-613.

Danzon P., Y.R. Wang and L. Wang (2003), "The impact of price regulation on the launch delay of new drugs. Evidence from twenty-five major markets in the 1990s," NBER Working Paper 9874.

David P. A. (1990), "The dynamo and the computer: an historical perspective on the modern productivity paradox," *The American Economic Review*, 80(2), 355-361.

David P. (1991), "Computer and Dynamo: The Modern Productivity Paradox in a not-too-Distant Mirror," in OECD, Paris: *Technology and Productivity: The Challenge for Economic Policy*.

Dean J. (1969), "Pricing Pioneering Products," *Journal of Industrial Economics*, 17, 165-179.

De Fabritiis G., F. Pammolli, M. Riccaboni (2003), "On Size and Growth of Business Firms," *Physica A*, 324(1-2), 38-44.

De la Dehesa G. (2006), *Europe at the Crossroads. Will the EU Ever be Able to Compete with the US as an Economic Power?*, New York: McGraw Hill.

de Mooij, Ruud A., and Sjef Ederveen (2003), "Taxation and Foreign Direct Investment: A Synthesis of Empirical Research," *International Tax and Public Finance* 10: 673-693.

Dincecco, M. (2006), "Fiscal Centralization, Limited Government, and Public Finances in Europe, 1650-1914," mimeo, IMT, Lucca.

Doms M.E. and J.B. Jensen (1998), "Comparing Wages, Skills and Productivity between Domestically and Foreign-Owned Manufacturing Establishments in the United States," in Lipsey R.E., R.E. Baldwin and J.D. Richardson, Eds., *Geography and Ownership as bases for Economic Accounting*, 235-258. University of Chicago.

Djankov, S. and P. Murrell (2002), "Enterprise Restructuring in Transition: a Quantitative Survey," *Journal of Economic Literature*, 40(3), 739-792.

Drabek Z. and J.C. Brada (1998), "Exchange Rate Regimes and the Stability of Trade Policy in Transition Economies," Staff Working Paper ERAD-98-07, World Trade Organization, Genéve.

Eaton J. and S. Kortum (2000), "Technology, Geography and Trade," working paper, Econ. Dept., Boston University.

EU Commission (2006a), "Price and Cost Competitiveness," EU, Brussels.

EU Commission (2006b), "Global Europe: Competing in the World," EU, Brussels.

EU Commission (2003), "The EU economy: 2003 review," EU, Brussels.

EUROSTAT (2004), "The Chemical Industry in the European Union," Statistics in Focus n.47, EU, Brussels.

EUROSTAT (2005), "The Pharmaceutical Industry in the European Union," Statistics in Focus n.44, EU, Brussels.

Evenett, S.J., and W. Keller (2002), "On Theories Explaining the Success of the Gravity Equation," *Journal of Political Economy*, 110(2), 281-316.

Evenson R.E. (1991), "Patent Data by Industry: Evidence for Invention Potential Exhaustion?" in *Technology and Productivity: The Challenge for Economic Policy*, 233-248, OECD, Paris.

Federal Trade Commission (2003), "To Promote Innovation: The Proper Balance of Competition and Patent Law and Policy."

Feenstra, R.C., Markusen, J.A., and A. K. Rose (1998), "Understanding the Home Market Effect and the Gravity Equation: The Role of Differentiating Goods," NBER Working Papers 6804, National Bureau of Economic Research, Inc.

Feenstra R.C., R. E. Lipsey, H. Deng, A. C. Ma, H. Mo (2005), "World Trade Flows: 1962-2000," NBER Working Paper 11040.

Feldstein M. (1995), "The Economics of Health and Health Care. What Have we Learned? What have I learned?" *American Economic Review Papers and Proceedings*, Vol. 85, n. 2, pp. 28-31.

Finn, M. G. (2003), "Stay rates of Foreign Doctorate Recipients from U.S. Universities," Oak Ridge, TN: Oak Ridge Institute for Science and Engineering.

Frankel, J.A. and A.K. Rose (2000), "Estimating the Effect of Currency Unions on Trade and Output," NBER Working Papers 7857.

Fu D., F. Pammolli, S.V. Buldyrev, M. Riccaboni, K. Yamasaki, K. Matia, H.E. Stanley (2005), "The Growth of Business Firms: Theoretical Framework and Empirical Evidence," *Proceedings of the National Academy of Sciences*, 102(52), 18801-6.

Federal Trade Commission (2003), "To Promote Innovation: the Proper Balance of Competition and Patent Law and Policy," Washington, DC.

GAO (1995), *Prescription Drug Prices: Official Index Overstates Producer Price Inflation*, United States General Accounting Office, GAO/HEHS-95-90, Washington D.C.

GOP (2000), Gambardella A., L. Orsenigo and F. Pammolli (2000), *Global Competitiveness in Pharmaceuticals: A European Perspective*, Directorate General Enterprise of the European Commission, November 2000.

Gomory, R. E. and W. J. Baumol (2001), *Global Trade and Conflicting National Interests*, Cambridge, MA: MIT Press.

Gordon R. (2000), "Does the 'New Economy' measure up to the great inventions of the past?" *The Journal of Economic Perspectives*, 14(4), 49-74.

Gordon R. (2002), "Technology and Economic Performance in the American Economy," Center for Economic Policy Research Discussion Paper 3213.

Gordon R. (2003), "Exploding Productivity Growth: Context, Causes, and Implications," Brookings Papers on Economic Activity, 2, 207-98.

Gordon R. (2004), "Why was Europe Left at the Station when America's Productivity Locomotive Departed?" NBER Working Paper 10661.

Griliches Z. (1957), "Hybrid Corn: An Exploration in the Economics of Technological Change," *Econometrica*, 25(4), 501-522.

Griliches Z. (1980), "Returns to Research and Development Expenditures in the Private Sector" in Kendrick J. and B. Vaccara (eds.), *New Development in Productivity Measurement and Analysis*, Chicago University Press, Chicago.

Griliches Z. (1984), *R&D, Patents and Productivity*, Chicago University Press.

Griliches Z. (1998), *R&D and Productivity: The Econometric Evidence*, Chicago University Press.

Griliches Z. and J. Mairesse (1983), "Comparing Productivity Growth: An Exploration of French and US Industrial and Firm Data," *European Economic Review*, 21, 89-119.

Groningen Growth and Development Centre, *60-Industry Database*, October 2005, http://www.ggdc.net.

Grossman G. and E. Rossi-Hansberg (2006), "Trading Tasks: A Simple Theory of Offshoring," August 2006. www.princeton.edu/~grossman/offshoring.pdf.

Grossman G. and E. Helpman (1991), *Innovation and Growth in the Global Economy*, Cambridge, MA: MIT Press.

Growiec J., Pammolli F., Riccaboni M. and H. E. Stanley (2007), "On the Size Distribution of Business Firms," *Economic Letters*, forthcoming.

Hall B. H. and J. Mairesse (1995), "Exploring the Relationship Between R&D and Productivity in French Manufacturing Firms," *Journal of Econometrics*, 65(1), 263-293.

Hege U., F. Palomino and A. Schwienbacher (2003), "Determinants of Venture Capital Performance: Europe and the United States," RICAFE working paper n. 1.

Helliwell J.F. (1998), *How Much Do National Borders Matter?* Brookings Institution, Washington DC.

Helpman E., and M. Trajtenberg (1998), "A Time to Sow and a Time to Reap: Growth Based on General Purpose Technologies" in Helpman, E. (ed.), *General Purpose Technologies and Economic Growth*, Cambridge, MA: MIT Press.

Helpman, E., (1987), ""Imperfect competition and international trade: Evidence from fourteen industrial countries," *Journal of the Japanese and International Economies*, 1(1), 62-81.

Helpman, E. (1999), "The Structure of Foreign Trade," *The Journal of Economic Perspectives*, 13(2), 121-144.

Helpman E., M. J. Melitz, and S. R. Yeaple (2004), "Export versus FDI with Heterogeneous Firms," *American Economic Review*, 94(1), 300-316.

Henderson R.M. and I.M. Cockburn (1996), "Scale, Scope, and Spillovers: Determinants of Research Productivity in the Pharmaceutical Industry," *RAND Journal of Economics*, 27(1), 32-59.

Hoffman J. (2005), "Generics Growth in the USA and the EU: The Role of India," *Journal of Generic Medicines*, 3(1), 7-19.

Hymer S. and P. Pashigian (1962), "Turnover of Firms As a Measure of Market Behavior," *The Review of Economics and Statistics*, 44(1), 82-87.

Ijiri Y. and H.A. Simon (1977), *Skew distributions and the sizes of business firms*, North Holland, New York.

Jeng L. and P. Wells (2000), "The Determinants of Venture Capital Funding: Evidence Across Countries," *Journal of Corporate Finance*, 6, 241-249.

Johnson, J. M. and M. Regets (1998), "International Mobility of Scientists and Engineers to the US—Brain Drain or Brain Circulation?" NSF Issue Brief 98-316.

Jones B.F. (2005), "The Burden of Knowledge and the 'Death of the Renaissance Man': Is Innovation Getting Harder?" NBER working paper 11360.

Jorgenson D. and Z. Grilliches (1967), "The Explanation of productivity change," *Review of Economic Studies*, 34, 249-283.

Jorgenson, D. (2001), "Information Technology and the U.S. Economy," *American Economic Review*, 91(1), 1-32.

Jorgenson, D., and Kun-Young Y. (2001), *Lifting the Burden: Tax Reform, the Cost of Capital, and U. S. Economic Growth*. Cambridge MA: MIT Press.

Jovanovic B. and P. L. Rousseau (2005), *General Purpose Technologies*, NBER working paper 11093.

Kanavos, P. (1998), "A Prospective View on European Pharmaceutical Research and Development. Policy Options to Reduce Fragmentation and Increase Competitiveness," *Pharmacoeconomics*, 13, 181-190.

Kanavos P., Costa-i-Font J., Merkur S., Gemmill M. (2004), *The Economic Impact of Pharmaceutical Parallel Trade in European Union Member States: A Stakeholder Analysis*, Special Research Paper, LSE Health and Social Care, London School of Economics and Political Science.

Kapur D., and J.McHale (2006), *Sojourns and software Internationally Mobilie Human Capital and High Tech Industry Development in India*, in Arora A. and A. Gambardella, Eds., *From Underdogs to Tigers*, Oxford University Press.

Kochhar, K., Kumar, U., Rajan, R., Subramanian, A. and I. Tokatlidis (2006), "India's pattern of development: What happened, what follows?" *Journal of Monetary Economics*, 53(5), 981-1019.

Kortum S. (1997), "Research, Patenting, and Technological Change," *Econometrica*, 65(6), 1389-1419.

Kortum S. and J. Lerner (2000), "Does Venture Capital Spur Innovation?" *Rand Journal of Economics*, 31, 674-692.

Kyle M. (2006), "Pharmaceutical Price Controls and Entry Strategies," *Review of Economics and Statistics*, forthcoming.

Lanjouw J.O. (2005), "Patents, Price Controls and Access to New Drugs: How Policy Affects Global Market Entry," NBER Working Paper 11321.

Lanjouw J.O. and I.M. Cockburn (2001), "New Pills for Poor People? Empirical Evidence after GATT," *World Development*, 29 (2), 265-289.

Leamer, E. E. and J.A. Levinsohn (1995), "International Trade Theory: The Evidence", in Grossman G. and K. Rogoff (eds), *Handbook of International Economics* Volume 3, Elsevier, North-Holland.

Lenz A.J. (2000), *The U.S. Current Account: A Sectoral Assessment of Performance and Prospects*, October 2000, report prepared for the U.S. Trade Deficit Review Commission, Washington DC.

Lerner, J. and R. Merges (1998), "The Control of Technology Alliances: An empirical Analysis of the Biotechnology Industry," *Journal of Industrial Economics*, 46(2), 125-156.

Lerner, J., Shane H. and Tsai A. (2003), "Do equity financing cycle matter? Evidence from biotechnology alliances," *Journal of Financial Economics*, 67, 411-446.

Levin R.C., A.K. Klevorick, R.R. Nelson, S.G. Winter, R. Gilbert, and Z. Griliches (1987), "Appropriating the Returns from Industrial Research and Development," *Brookings Papers on Economic Activity*, 3, 783-831, The Brookings Institution.

Linder S. (1961), *An Essay on Trade and Transformation*, New York: John Wiley.

Lichtenberg F.R. (2003), "The impact of new drug launches on longevity: evidence from longitudinal disease-level data from 52 countries, 1982-2001," NBER working paper n. 9754.

Lichtenberg F. and D. Siegel (1991), "The Impact of R&D investment on Productivity: New Evidence using R&D-LRD Data," *Economic Inquiry*, 29(2), 203-228.

Lichtenberg F.R. and J.Waldfogel (2003), "Does Misery love Company? Evidence from Pharmaceutical markets before and after the Orphan drug Act,", NBER Working Paper 9750.

Lipsey R., and M.Y. Weiss (1981), "Foreign Production and Exports in Manufacturing Industries," *Review of Economics and Statistics*, 63(4), 488-494.

Lööf H. and A. Heshmati (2001), "Knowledge Capital and Performance Heterogeneity: A Firm Level Innovation Study," *International Journal of Production Economics*, 76(1), 61-85.

Lu, Z.J. and W.S. Comanor (1998), "Strategic Pricing of New Pharmaceuticals," *The Review of Economics and Statistics*, 80 (1), 108-118.

Magazzini L., F. Pammolli, M. Riccaboni (2004), "Dynamic Competition in Pharmaceuticals: On Patent Expiry, Generic Penetration and Industry Structure," *European Journal of Health Economics*, 5, 175-182.

Mansfield E. (1986), "Patents and Innovation: An Empirical Study," *Management Science*, 32 (2) 173-181.

McCallum, J. (1995), "National Borders Matter: Canada-U.S. Regional Trade Patterns," *American Economic Review*, 85(3), 615-623.

McKinsey Global Institute (2001), "U.S. productivity growth 1995-2000, Understanding the contribution of Information Technology relative to other factors."

MERIT (2003), "Brain Drain—Emigration Flows for Qualified Scientists," report of the European project for the Competitiveness, Economic Analysis and Indicators Unit of the Directorate for the Knowledge-based economy and society of the Directorate General for Research, UNU-Merit, Maastricht.

Mervis J. (2005), "Productivity Counts—But the definition is key," *Science*, 309(29) July 2005.

Mintz J.M., Chen D., Guillemette Y., Poschmann F. (2005), *The 2005 Tax Competitiveness Report: Unleashing the Canadian Tiger*, C.D. Howe Institute, n. 216, www.cdhowe.org

Mossialos, E., Mrazek, M. and T. Walley, Eds. (2004), "Regulating Pharmaceuticals in Europe: Striving for Efficiency, Equity and Quality," Open University Press, Maidenhead, Berkshire (UK).

Munos B. (2006), "Can Open-Source R&D Reinvigorate Drug Research?" *Nature Reviews Drug Discovery*, 5(9), 723-729.

Nordhaus W. (2001), "Productivity Growth and the New Economy," NBER Working Paper 8096.

O'Mahony M., and B. van Ark (2003), *EU productivity and competitiveness: An industry perspective. Can Europe resume the catching-up process?* European Commission, Brussels.

OECD (2001), *Competition and regulation issues in the pharmaceutical industry*, Directorate for Financial, Fiscal and Enterprise Affairs, OECD Paris.

OECD (2003), *OECD Science, Technology and Industry Scoreboard*, OECD, Paris.

OECD (2004), *ANBERD database*, OECD, Paris.

OECD (2004a), *Main Economic Indicators Database*, OECD, Paris.

OECD (2004b), *STAN Industry Database*, OECD, Paris.

OECD (2005a), *OECD Health Data 2005*, OECD, Paris.

OECD (2005b), *Measuring Globalization OECD Economic Globalization Indicators*, vol. 2005, no. 39, OECD, Paris.

Oliner S., and D. Sichel (2000), "The Resurgence of Growth in the Late 1990s: Is Information Technology the Story?" *Journal of Economic Perspectives*, 14(4), 3-22.

Orsenigo L., F. Pammolli, and M. Riccaboni (2001), "Technological Change and Network Dynamics. Lessons from the Pharmaceutical Industry," *Research Policy*, 30(3), 485-508.

Owen-Smith J., M. Riccaboni, F. Pammolli, and W.W. Powell (2002), "A Comparison of U.S. and European University-Industry Relations in the Life Sciences," *Management Sciences*, 48(1), 24-43.

Pammolli F. and M. Riccaboni (2004), "Market Structure and Drug Innovation," *Health Affairs*, 23(1), 48-50.

Pammolli F., L. Magazzini, and L. Orsenigo (2002), "The Intensity of Competition after Patent Expiry in Pharmaceuticals: A Cross-Country Analysis," *Revue of Economie Industrielle*, 99, 107-132.

Pammolli F., Nicita A., Riccaboni M., Baio G., and L. Magazzini (2002), *The Italian Decree DL 15/04/2002, no. 63 on Pharmaceutical Expenditure Containment: Impact on Industry and Market Distortions.* Mimeo, University of Florence

Pammolli F., M. Riccaboni and L. Orsenigo (2000), "Variety and Irreversibility in Scientific and Technological Systems," in Nicita A. and U. Pagano, eds., *The Evolution of Economic Diversity*, Routledge, London, UK.

Pammolli F., and N.C. Salerno (2006), "Public finances sustainability, structural reforms, and health spending in Europe," *CERM working paper*, mimeo.

Phelps E. (2003), "Economic underperformance in Continental Europe: A prospering Economy Runs on the Dynamism from its Economic Institutions," lecture, Royal Institute for International Affairs, London, March 18.

Porter M.E. (1985), *Competitive Advantage*, Free Press, New York.

Porter M.E. (1990), "The Competitive Advantage of Nations," Harvard Business Review, (March/April 1990), 73-91.

Powell W.W., K.W. Koput, L. Smith-Doer (1996), "Interorganizational Collaboration and the Locus of Innovation: Networks of Learning in Biotechnology," *Administrative Science Quarterly*, 41 (1), 116-145.

Prescott, E. (2004), "Why do Americans work so much more than Europeans?" *Quarterly Review*, Federal Reserve Bank of Minneapolis, July, 2-13.

Rabinow P. (1997), *Making PCR: A Story of Biotechnology*, University of Chicago Press, Chicago.

Reekie, W.D. (1978), "Price and Quality Competition in the United States Drug Industry," *Journal of Industrial Economics*, Vol. 26, 223-237.

Rodrik, D. (2006), "What's So Special About China's Exports?" *China and the World Economy*, forthcoming.

Rodrik, D. and A. Subramanian (2004), "From "Hindu Growth" to Productivity Surge: The Mystery of the Indian Growth Transition," *IMF Working Papers* 04/77, International Monetary Fund.

Roland G. (1989), *Economie Politique du Systhéme Sovietique*, L'Harmattan, Paris.

Romer P. M. (1990), "Endogenous Technological Change," *Journal of Political Economy*, 98(5), S71-S102.

Saxenian, A. (2005), "From Brain Drain to Brain Circulation: Transnational Communities and Regional Upgrading in India and China," *Studies in Comparative International Development*, 40(2), 35-61.

Schmookler J. (1966), *Invention and Economic Growth*, Harvard University Press Cambridge, MA.

Segerstrom P. (1998), "Endogenous Growth Without Scale Effects," *American Economic Review*, December 1998, 88(5), 1290-1310.

Shapiro, C. (1983), "Optimal Pricing of Experience Goods," Bell Journal of Economics, 14, 497-507.

Smith A. (1986), *An Inquiry into the Nature and Causes of the Wealth of Nations*. Penguin Books, Harmondsworth, UK (first published 1776).

Sullivan, Martin A., "Latest IRS Data Show Jump in Tax Haven Profits," *Tax Notes*, October 11, 2004.

Sutton J. (1998), *Technology and Market Structure*, Cambridge MA: MIT Press,

Thurow, L. C. (1992), *Head to Head: The Coming Economic Battle Among Japan, Europe, and America*, St. Leonards, NSW: Allen & Unwin.

Tinbergen J. (1962), *Shaping the World Economy*, Twentieth Century Fund, New York.

Toole, A.A. (2000), "The Impact of Public Basic Research on Industrial Innovation: Evidence from the Pharmaceutical Industry," *SIEPR Discussion Paper*, 00-07, Stanford University, CA.

Trefler D. (1995), "The Case of Missing Trade and Other Mysteries," *American Economic Review*, 85(5), 1029-1046.

Vernon R. (1966), "International Investment and International Trade in the Product Cycle," *Quarterly Journal of Economics*, 80 (May 1966), 190-207.

Vernon, J.M. (1971), "Concentration, Promotion, and Market Share Stability in the Pharmaceutical Industry," *The Journal of Industrial Economics*, 19(3), 246-266.

UNCTAD (2006), *World Investment Report*, United Nations, New York and Geneva.

U.S. Department of Commerce (2004), *Manufacturing in America: A Comprehensive Strategy to Address the Challenges to U.S. Manufacturers*, U.S. Government Printing Office, Washington DC.

U.S. Senate Finance Committee (1996), Final Report from the Advisory Committee To Study The Consumer Price Index, U.S. Government Printing Office, Washington DC.

USITC (1998), *Shifts in U.S. Merchandise Trade in 1997*, U.S. International Trade Commission, Investigation No. 332-345, Publication 3120, Washington DC.

USITC (1999) "Outsourcing by the Pharmaceutical Industry Provides Opportunities for Fine Chemical Producers Worldwide," *Industry Trade and Technology Review*, 3253, Oct. 1999, pp 1-14.

USITC (2001), *Shifts in U.S. Merchandise Trade in 2000*, U.S. International Trade Commission, Investigation No. 332-345, Publication 3436, Washington DC.

USITC (2005), *Shifts in U.S. Merchandise Trade in 2004*, U.S. International Trade Commission, Investigation No. 332-345, Publication 3789, Washington DC.

Weisbrod, B. (1991), "The Health Care Quadrilemma: An Essay on Technological Change, Insurance, Quality of Care, and Cost Containment," *Journal of Economic Literature*, 29(2), 523-52.

Weston J.F. (1979), "Pricing in the Pharmaceutical Industry," in R.I. Chien, Eds., *Issues in Pharmaceutical Economics*, Lexington , MA.

Weston J.F. (1982), "A Survey of the Economics of the Pharmaceutical Industry with Emphasis on Economic Factors in Price Differentials," in *The effectiveness of Medicines in Containing Dental Care Costs: Impact of Innovation, Regulation, and Quality*, Washington, DC.

Yang S., and E. Brynjolfsson (2001), "Intangible Assets and Growth Accounting: Evidence from Computer Investments," MIT Working Paper 136.

About the Authors

Fabio Pammolli is Director of the IMT Lucca Institute for Advanced Studies and a Professor of Economics and Management at the University of Florence. His research interests are in the fields of economics of innovation, industrial dynamics and market regulation, processes of industrial growth in markets and networks, economic analysis of the pharmaceutical industry. He is the author of many publications. He is a former Member of the Commission on Intellectual Property Rights, Innovation and Public Health at the World Health Organization in Geneva; Director of European Pharmaceutical Innovation and Regulation Systems; and President of CERM, Center for the Economic Analysis of Competitiveness, Markets and Regulation.

Massimo Riccaboni is Associate Professor of Economics and Management at the University of Florence and a Senior Research Fellow of CERM, Center for the Economic Analysis of Competitiveness, Markets and Regulation. His research interests are in the fields of economics of innovation, industrial dynamics, processes of industrial growth in markets and networks, and economic analysis of the pharmaceutical industry. He has published in, among others, *The Proceedings of the National Academy of Sciences, The Journal of the European Economics Association, The International Journal of Industrial Organization, Management Science, Economics Letters, Health Affairs,* and *E. Journal of Health Economics.*